MAKE-UP MADE EASY

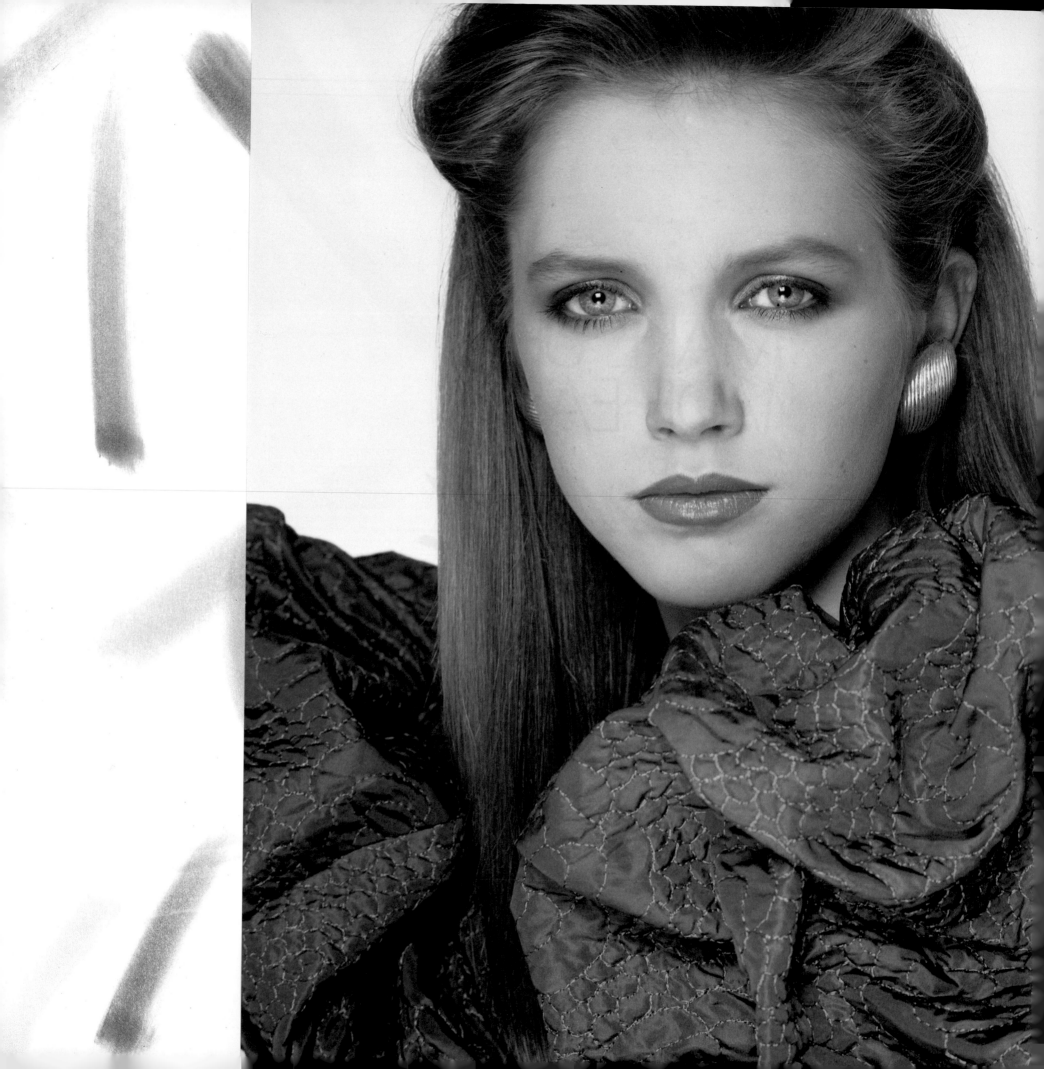

CONTENTS

Introduction	7
Skin Care	9
Your Skin Type	10
Skin Care Routine	12
Give Yourself a Facial	14
Face Masks	16
Skin and the Elements	18
Body Care	20
Hand Care	22
Foot Care	24
Eyebrows	26
Salon Services	27
Make-up	29
Foundation	30
Concealers, Blushers, Powder	32
Face Shapes	34
Square Face	34
Round Face	35
Long Face	36

Eyes	38
Blue Eyes	40
Brown Eyes	44
Green Eyes	48
Grey Eyes	52
Eye Care	57
Lips	59
Lip Colours	61
Lip Shapes	61
Looks for Lifestyles	64
Difficult Colours	64
Understated Make-up	66
A Party Piece	68
Look for Day	70
Look for Night	72
What's Best for Black?	74
Quick Face	76
What's Right for White?	78
Index	80

First published in Great Britain in 1984 by
Artus Publishing Company Ltd

This edition published in 1989 by
Treasure Press
Michelin House
81 Fulham Road
London SW3 6RB

Reprinted 1990

Copyright © Barbara Daly 1984

ISBN 1 85051 418 6

Produced by Mandarin Offset
Printed and bound in Hong Kong

Photography by
John Swannell

Hair by Nicky Clark and
Melanie Taylor at John Frieda

Fashion editor Annabel Hodin
Styling Elspeth Norden

Illustrations by John Babbage

Design and art direction by
Nick Overhead

Edited by Sue Cooper

A facial every six to eight weeks, or monthly if skin is oily will deep cleanse your skin. You can get a professional facial in a salon, or do a basic steam treatment quite easily in your own home.

Heat is one of the most important factors of a facial – it softens and slightly opens the pores so that the cleansing agents can do their job really well. Steam oily skins for 3 to 4 minutes, but give dry skins 7 to 8 minutes. They require more moisture to soften the skin, whereas oily skin is already rather more lubricated – with its own oil.

Home facials are suitable for all skin types, only the routine changes according to your skin type. Choose a time of day when you won't need to apply make-up for several hours. First make sure all your hair is tied well back off your face. Don't wear anything with a high neck. A towel wrapped around your top half, or a dressing gown with the collar turned back will enable you to cleanse right to the collar bone.

Have all your equipment laid out and ready on a tray. This will include – cleanser and eye make-up remover; eyebrow tweezers and a magnifying mirror; an antiseptic solution; creams for massaging into the face; a face mask according to your skin type; and a light moisturiser. Cotton wool and tissues will be needed, and last, but not least, a large bowl of hot water, a towel and a few fragrant herbs, such as rosemary or peppermint. These aren't essential, but they make the water smell sweet, and the aromatic vapours help clear your nose.

THE ROUTINE

1 Cleanse face, as before (see page 12).
2 Steam face for 3 to 4 minutes if oily; 7 to 8 minutes if dry. Pour hot water into the basin, toss in your herbs and drape a towel over your head. Bend over the water, being careful not to let the hot water touch your face. You don't have to be very far down over the steam – just a waft of it is enough. There's no need to come out looking beetroot red.
3 Once you've steamed your face thoroughly:
If treating *dry skin* . . .
Inspect it closely in the magnifying mirror for blackheads around the nose and chin that could be easily removed now that the skin is warm and soft. Do so by covering the fingertips with tissue, and squeezing gently (see page 13). If the blackhead doesn't come out easily, leave it alone. Dab the area with antiseptic.
If treating *oily skin* . . .
This skin may be spotty – now's the time to try and get rid of some of the spots. Dab the infected areas very lightly with antiseptic, cover your fingertips with tissue, and squeeze blackheads, spots and pimples very gently. They

should pop out quite easily now the skin is soft and warm. Be gentle – do only what is easy, and not all in one go. Dab all areas that have been squeezed with antiseptic.
4 All skin types will now need a very light massage to reduce redness and give an even skin tone. Massage helps bring the blood to the surface of the skin, giving you a healthy glow. If your skin is dry choose a rich treatment cream or oil – put a dollop of it in the palm of your hand to warm it up. Dot all over the face and neck, and starting at the base of the neck massage in small upward circular movements from the collar-bone to the chin and face, and right up to the hairline. Be careful around the eye area – don't pull.

If your skin is oily use a treatment cream suitable for your skin type, or a very small amount of moisturiser – just enough to allow your fingertips to slide over the surface of the skin without dragging.

5 Carefully remove all the skin cream with cotton wool dampened in warm water. You'll be amazed at how much dirt will continue to come out of the skin, even though you've cleansed it. Don't forget to wipe over the neck, hairline, and side of the face very thoroughly.
6 Now's the time to pluck your eyebrows. The hair should come out easily because the skin is warm and soft, and the cleanness reduces any risk of infection as the hair comes out cleanly from the root. (See page 26 for how to do this.)
7 Next apply a face mask and relax. (On the next page I'll tell you how to choose and use a face mask.) Finish with your regular moisturiser.

GIVE YOURSELF A FACIAL

However good your daily cleansing routine, a once-in-a-while deep cleanse, or facial, will rout out all traces of grime and grease, make spots, blackheads and pimples less likely, and give you time to yourself to relax!

Masks can be softening and soothing, or firming and stimulating, depending on which one you choose

Your particular skin type may need *two* different kinds of mask, on different areas of the face; i.e. a mask for dry skin on cheeks and throat, and another for greasy skin on the T-zone. You may also prefer different types of face mask at different times of the year. In winter something which softens and stimulates your skin may be better than the cooling and toning type you would choose for the summer.

Always read labels carefully, to make sure you are getting the right one for your skin type. Their colour is often a rough guide – but you can't always see it, or rely on it!

Clay-Based Masks: (usually white or off-white in colour) are best for oily skins. They dry on the skin, sometimes going quite hard, and at the same time absorb excess oil and draw out impurities. Rinse off the mask and the oil and impurities are washed away too! Because of their drying property, though, clay masks should not be used on the neck or around the delicate eye area, and, for the same reason, it's not a good idea to use them more than once a week.

Fruit, Vegetable or Herb Masks: are very common, and available for oily, dry or normal skins, depending on what type of base they have – clay or cream. The clay ones work with the same 'drawing and absorbing' action as described above. The cream-based ones are usually more moisturising, containing a higher fat content to keep the skin soft. They, like all masks, give a deep cleansing treatment, and the addition of the various fruit, vegetable or herb extracts is either to soften, soothe, or stimulate the surface of the skin according to its type. There are also cream masks which have especially gentle formulations for sensitive skins.

These masks will usually be tinted according to the extract they contain. The astringent ones for oily skin will often be blue or green. The fruity ones for normal to dry skin are often peach or pink. These don't dry on the skin and they usually have to be tissued off as well as rinsed with warm water. Some of the gentler masks can be applied over the eyes and most of them should be applied to the neck as well as the face. They can be used once a week or more often if necessary.

Oil-Based Masks: are designed for very dry skins. More oil can be absorbed from a mask than from an ordinary moisturiser, since it's applied to the skin after cleansing and during a facial. The skin is warm and receptive to the softening oil, which is left on the face for 10 to 15 minutes.

Some oil-based masks contain added ingredients, such as herbs, egg or honey, and they tend to be cream, or yellow in colour – or occasionally pale pink.

Gel Masks: are for oily to normal or dry skins. They're very good for gentle exfoliating, because when they are removed the peeling process removes the dead surface of the skin, leaving the skin looking fresh and more translucent.

They're never to be used around the eyes because they pull the skin slightly as they are removed, and for the same reason you have to be careful not to apply the gel too thickly, or too close to the hairline. It can stick to your hair and be difficult and painful to remove. Gel masks, again, depend on your skin type for extract ingredients, and hence, colour – but they will always be transparent.

FACE MASKS FROM THE FRIDGE

If you feel in need of a real face treat but don't have a face mask to hand, take a look around your kitchen. You'll probably find all the ingredients for a home-made mask to suit all skin types. Use quickly, as they don't keep.

Cucumber Mask
$\frac{1}{2}$ cup cucumber pieces (including peel)
1 egg white
1 tablespoon dry milk powder
Put all the ingredients into a blender and process at high speed until smooth. Apply to face with cotton pad and allow to remain on 15 to 20 minutes. Remove with lukewarm water.

Honey and Oatmeal Mask
1 fresh egg yolk
1 teaspoon olive oil
3–4 drops lemon juice
$\frac{1}{4}$ teaspoon honey
$\frac{1}{2}$ teaspoon plain uncooked oatmeal (porridge oats)
$\frac{1}{2}$ teaspoon powdered milk
$\frac{1}{2}$ teaspoon powdered laundry starch
Mix the ingredients together. Smooth over face with fingertips. Leave on for 10 minutes if skin is dry, 15 minutes if skin is normal, and 20 minutes if skin is oily. Rinse off with lukewarm water. Splash with invigorating cold water. Pat dry.

FACE MASKS

Take off a face mask and you take with it a layer of dead, dry skin cells that could be clouding your skin – making it dull. You get a glow, and a deep cleanse with it, that's an integral part of any facial.

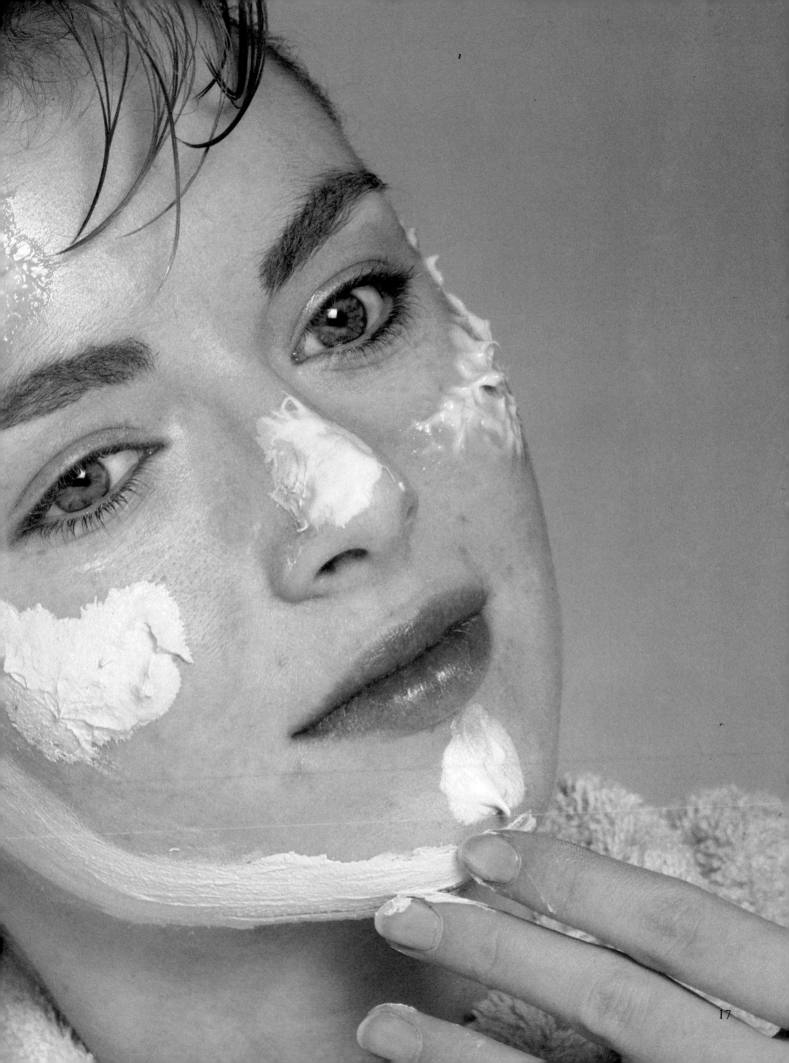

Protection is the key to supple, clear, and healthy skin. However well you look after your skin throughout your life it will age as you grow older. It's a natural process and one that, to date, science has found no way of stopping. But this doesn't mean it has to be a harsh ageing process. Any age group can have a healthy-looking skin, and, even if at fifty some wrinkles are inevitable, your skin will still look good if you've taken care of it from an early age.

HARSH WEATHER

One thing that causes the skin to get rougher and harder is harsh weather – cold wind and rain can both speed up the evaporation of your skin's own water, leaving it dry. The best protection you can get is a good moisturiser – and a lip cream or stick. Moisturisers work by laying a fine film of oil over the surface of your skin to prevent evaporation of your skin's own moisture (see page 10). The oil literally 'seals in' your skin's water – preventing dryness and cracking. In winter you need a very occlusive or 'sealing' cream – a cold-cream-type formula – as humidity is low and there is less moisture in the air.

In summer, when it's hot and humidity is high, you can change to a lighter moisturiser. Now that your skin may be hot and sweating, you need a formula that will allow air to get to your skin – sealing in some of your skin's moisture, but allowing perspiration to escape. Lotions, or light greaseless creams leave a 'patchy' film over your skin, rather than an all-over seal.

Make-up helps form a barrier against the elements too. Choose a moisturised foundation, and a creamy lipstick, which should be re-applied often. Lips dry out just as quickly as the skin on your face, so protect them with a lip-salve when not wearing lipstick in winter, and with a total sun-block stick in summer or hot sunshine.

If the elements are really harsh, don't think twice about wrapping your face in a scarf, wearing a hat or a veil, or anything you fancy to create a layer between you and the weather outdoors.

Don't worry too much about rain, however. Contrary to popular belief, as long as it's not coupled with biting winds, rain doesn't harm the skin. Remember, though, if your face gets very wet – dab it dry, cleanse and put on a fresh layer of moisturiser!

CITY LIVING

Indoors, there's air conditioning, central heating, and dry office atmospheres; outdoors, there's all the grime, dust and fumes that city pollution can throw at you – so how can your skin cope? Dirt gives your skin a dull, lacklustre appearance, in itself very ageing, so in the city cleansing becomes doubly important. Apart from being extra particular about your skin care routine (see page 12), exfoliation can help to clear away that dull look. Creams which contain tiny granules are massaged gently over the skin for about 30 seconds – avoiding the delicate eye and lip areas. The grains slough off the surface layer of dead skin cells, and with it ingrained grime, grease and flaky rough skin. Some exfoliative creams contain synthetic particles of polyethylene – others are made granular by natural products, such as crushed apricot shells.

Use them once a week if skin is oily or dry – and only when skin needs a 'pep up' if you're at all sensitive.

Beat dryness indoors with a good occlusive moisturiser – spray your face with mineral water, then apply your cream for maximum effect. Try to raise the humidity in air-conditioned offices with a few bowls of water placed around – or with a humidifier machine.

SUN PROTECTION

Deep, dark tans are a status symbol of the past! Now the message has reached most of us that long unprotected spells in the sun mean a bigger risk of wrinkles. The aim should be a more subtle, golden glow – achieved with the careful use of suntan creams and lotions.

Look for the Sun-Protection Factor – the number on your sun cream. If you can normally stay in the sun for 10 minutes with no cream before burning, you'll be able to spend 60 minutes in the sun with a factor 6 cream, i.e. 6 times as long! Take several sun factors on holiday with you. Start by using the highest number for the first few days, and gradually work your way down. Your skin will build its own resistance to the sun as it tans – so by the end of the holiday you'll be able to use quite a low-factor cream.

If you are very fair, or just don't want to tan at all, use a product which says it is a Total Sun Block. It's a good idea to have a total-sun-block stick for eyelids, nose and lips anyway.

Young skins that are suffering from oiliness may find the sun helpfully drying – and it's known that ultraviolet light helps acne – but they still need protection from the *burning* rays of the sun, with frequent applications of sun cream.

SKIN AND THE ELEMENTS

Sun, wind, pollution and the atmosphere you live in can affect your skin just as much as any creams or lotions you put on it. It is proven beyond all shadow of a doubt that excessive sun helps to age the skin prematurely, and harsh weather, wind, central heating, air conditioning, and general neglect all need to be guarded against by taking proper care of the skin.

BODY CARE

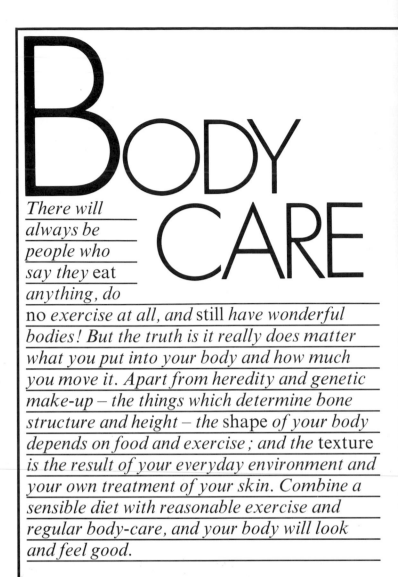

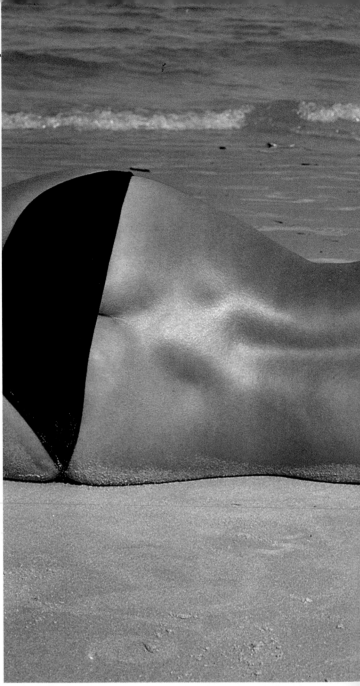

There will always be people who say they eat anything, do no *exercise at all, and* still *have wonderful bodies! But the truth is it really does matter what you put into your body and how much you move it. Apart from heredity and genetic make-up – the things which determine bone structure and height – the* shape *of your body depends on food and exercise; and the* texture *is the result of your everyday environment and your own treatment of your skin. Combine a sensible diet with reasonable exercise and regular body-care, and your body will look and feel good.*

WHAT YOU EAT

What you eat keeps you healthy, and thoughts on nutrition are updated regularly as more is learned about the effects of food on our bodies. We now know that we don't need vast amounts of protein and fat to grow and be strong – the emphasis has shifted towards eating more fibre and starchy carbohydrate for a healthy diet.

You may think it's difficult to alter the eating habits of a lifetime, and, of course, you must take into account your individual tastes, how you live, and what you can afford. But there are some simple ways of changing your day-to-day diet for the better.

Moderation in all things is very important – too much of anything is a bad thing. You can make yourself just as unhealthy on carrot juice as you can on sugary drinks, if you overdose on either. Ideally a good rounded diet should include less fat, less sugar, less salt, but more starchy

carbohydrate and more fibre.

Cut down or avoid obviously sugary and fatty foods, such as cakes, sweets, fats and fatty meats, but try to eat more fruit, vegetables, cereals and whole grains. Make *some* of your breakfast toast out of 100 per cent wholemeal bread, or at least substitute it for the white bread on alternate days. Instead of eating sugar-coated cereals, have high-fibre home-made muesli, whole-wheat cereal, or porridge. Try and develop a taste for unsweetened drinks and food. Cut your white sugar by half in tea and coffee, then gradually try to go without it. Use semi-skimmed or skimmed milk instead of full-fat milk, or for cereals try unsweetened fruit juice, or low fat yoghurt as delicious alternatives.

Buy margarines which are labelled 'high in poly-unsaturates', instead of butter. And remember, cheese may be a delicious snack, or decorative topping, but it is also high in protein and fat, so don't

discount it when looking at your protein intake. If you love cheese, pick a low-fat type, such as Edam, Brie, or cottage cheese, rather than a high-fat Cheddar or Stilton.

Fruit and vegetables contain fibre and vitamins. Eat at least one piece of citrus fruit a day, such as a grapefruit or orange – it's a tasty alternative to a Vitamin C pill. The whole fruit is more filling and better for you than a glass of fruit juice.

Roughage and protein abound in all the beans, peas and lentils available. There are lots of ways of using them, apart from merely putting them in stews and soups.

If you want to avoid consuming large amounts of preservative, additives, sugars, salt, and colouring, try not to eat too many processed,

canned, pre-packed foodstuffs. This doesn't include wrapped fresh foods. If you do buy cans (and which of us doesn't), get into the habit of reading the labels carefully. Choose fruits canned in natural juice rather than in sugary syrup. Look for vegetables which are packed with 'no added salt', and for fish packed in brine, rather than oil. Many of the frozen foods are frozen with no additives at all. But, of course, it's better to go for fresh foodstuffs wherever possible. It is true – you are what you eat!

HOW YOU MOVE

How you move keeps your body supple and in shape. Exercise is essential. That doesn't mean you have to go to a keep-fit class, or take up jogging, or a strenuous sport,

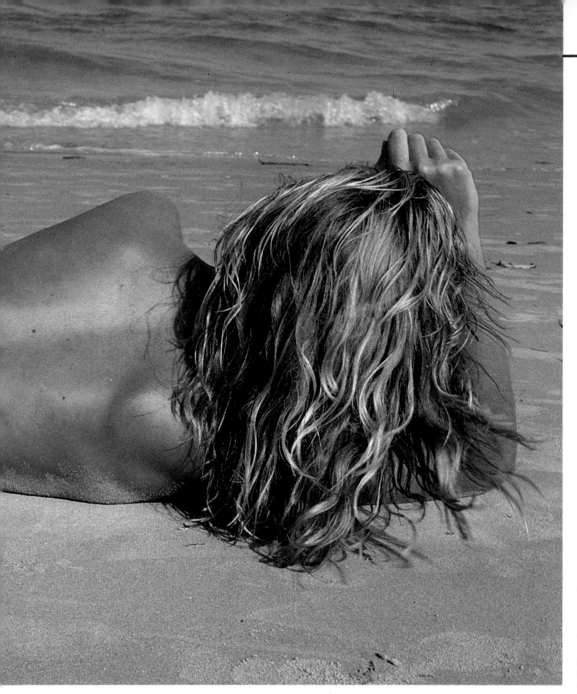

although all or any one of these things is a good idea if you feel like it. Exercise means keeping your body on the move for a certain amount of time each day. The movement of your body should include something that makes your pulse race, your heart beat faster and your blood circulate rapidly. Walking briskly or going up and down stairs for 10 minutes will do just this; taking a 10-minute run or jog is even better. Exercise should also include movements that stretch and strengthen the muscles – swimming is one of the best, as are most sports and any vigorous dancing. Our bodies don't work at their best if we just sit or lie around during our waking hours – to keep them supple, strong and healthy we need to keep them exercised.

Apart from toning the muscles, exercise is an important way of relieving stress and tiredness. Get yourself moving, and it's known that the body produces hormones which lift your mood – give you a sort of high! Even when you're tired after a day in a stuffy workplace, exercise will change that lethargic type of fatigue into a feeling of refreshed relaxation. As you build up your stamina you also build up your energy level – so the fitter you are the more energy you have to enjoy life.

Exercise also helps you look good! It increases circulation and blood flow to the skin, giving you a glow. And it helps burn off calories – so if you're deciding to lose a bit of weight you can speed up the process by exercising regularly.

HOW YOU CARE FOR YOUR BODY

How you care for your body on the outside decides your skin's texture. Skin is the same all over the body and needs just as much attention, say, on your knees and elbows, as on your face. It may be thicker and thinner in certain areas, thinner on cheeks, thicker on legs, for instance, but it can still be dry or oily – or have dry or oily patches – just as on the face. You may have an oily back, but dry arms and legs, so take this into account when planning your body care. If you do have oily patches, avoid using bath oils, body lotions or fatty soaps. Keep those areas scrupulously clean with a mild soap and water, and be careful not to let long hair or falling dandruff irritate any spotty skin. You can treat spots, pimples and blackheads the same as you would on your face (see page 13), but it's better to leave them alone.

For most people the biggest problem with body skin is dryness. The areas of your body that take pressure, your hands, elbows and feet, for example, build up layers of rough skin. Regular exfoliating, with a granular body cream, pumice stone, or simple coarse salt, will help to smooth them – and stop upper arms getting goose-fleshy.

If the rest of your body feels dry use bath oil, moisturising bath foams, or even baby oil in your bath water. Bath salts and foaming bubble baths are more drying, but you can off-set this by *always* rubbing body lotion all over as soon as you've dried yourself after the bath. Buy large economy-size body lotions – you'll get through a lot of them!

Unless you do a job which causes all your body skin to become grimy, it isn't usually necessary to soap the entire body, even though you wash it every day. Instead, soap just the back if oily, and don't bother to soap tummy, chest, arms and legs. Not using too much soap will help your body retain some of its natural oils, essential for a healthy skin. Over-washing can cause dry patches, flakiness and sores.

Deodorants are important depending on the amount you perspire. Some people need only a light deodorant/anti-perspirant for their underarms, while others need a stronger anti-perspirant, especially in the summer months. All deodorants and anti-perspirants work best on hair-free skin. Although there are various kinds of body deodorants on the market, they are neither necessary, nor particularly useful. Regular washing and a light dusting of talcum powder is enough to keep everybody fresh and sweet. Remember, too, that natural fibres, such as pure cotton, or wool and cotton mixed, absorb moisture better than artificial fabrics. So if you have a perspiration problem try to avoid wearing synthetics as much as possible.

HAND CARE

Hands work even harder than our faces! They're constantly out in all weather, plunging into water and diving into detergents, yet so often we deny them the care they're due. They need just as much attention as our complexions.

Protect your hands as much as possible – they can quickly show signs of wear, tear, and ageing. Wear barrier cream, outdoor gloves when in bad weather, and household gloves when working indoors. Use hand cream as often as possible – get into the habit of applying it every time you dry your hands.

Exercise your hands to keep them supple, and reduce the risk of arthritic fingers in later years. Stretch out your arms and make a tight fist; then fling your fingers outwards a couple of times. Circle your hands from the wrist, and shake them about to get the circulation moving.

Once you've started this basic care and protection your fingernails will automatically improve (unless you're a nail-biter!), but there are some problems, such as flaking and brittle nails, that can be helped with a good manicure.

THE MANICURE

Start by collecting together the things you'll need . . .
A small bowl of warm water (a sponge is nice to press on)
An emery board or nail file
An orange stick – with cotton wool wrapped around the tip
Cuticle clippers
Nail polish remover
Cuticle cream and cuticle remover
Hand cream
Nail polish – including base coat and hardener.

1 Remove old nail polish.
2 File the nail into shape – not too pointed, and not filed too far down at the sides. File in *one* direction only, from the side to the tip – not back and forth. Round off the top to a shape somewhere between an oval and a square.
3 Massage a dot of cuticle cream into each nail and dip fingers in water for 2 minutes.
4 Dab hands dry. Ease back cuticle with your cotton-wool-tipped orange stick. Use little circular movements.
5 If you have a lot of skin clinging to the nail bed, use a cuticle remover. Wipe off the cuticle cream and paint cuticle remover around each nail bed. Work around the cuticle again with fresh cotton wool on your orange stick.
6 Wash off cuticle remover. Dry your hands.
7 If you have loose skin or hang nails around the edges of your nails snip away with cuticle clippers. *Never cut around the whole cuticle* – the skin grows back into a hard horny layer. Clippers are extremely sharp so be careful not to slip.
8 Massage a generous dollop of hand cream from fingertips to elbows!
9 Make sure there's no cream left on your nails. Apply base coat, as you would any polish. This gives a good finish and stops dark-coloured nail polishes from staining the nails.
10 When dry apply nail polish. Starting with the little finger, paint a semicircle of polish close to the cuticle, leaving a hair's width between polish and cuticle. Paint the centre of the nail, then each side. Most polishes need two or three coats. Allow each coat to dry for several minutes before applying the next, otherwise the polish stays soft and chips.
11 Top the nail polish with a coat of sealer to harden the surface and hold the gloss. If you don't like coloured nail polish use a base coat by itself, or with a transparent polish, or simply buff the nails.

NAIL PROBLEMS

Stained Nails or Fingers
Remove stains with a drop of lemon juice, or hydrogen peroxide. Rinse the nails well and apply hand cream.

Flaking Nails
Cutting nails with scissors puts a strain on the nail bed. This can cause the nail layers to split and separate. Keep flaking nails short, buff often, and use a nail hardener and cuticle cream regularly.

Brittle Nails
Treat these in the same way as flaking nails. Include lots of foods rich in Vitamin B in your diet for both – e.g. liver and green vegetables. Avoid anything which will dry your nails; wear rubber gloves whenever using water.

White Flecks
These indicate damage to the nail bed under the skin. You may have knocked your nail. Camouflage with nail polish.

Ridges
Ridges can be the result of damage to the nail bed, rough treatment, or illness. Ridge fillers are available. Paint on before polish to give nails a smooth surface

Weak Nails
Reinforce with brush-on liquid fibre nail strengtheners, which coat the nail with a criss-cross of artificial fibres. Protect your nails and eat a varied diet and you should not have too many problems.

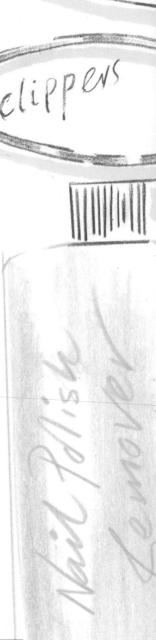

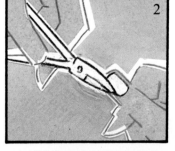

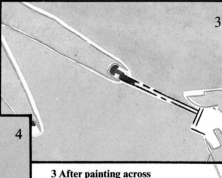

1 Ease back cuticles with a cotton-wool-tipped orange stick, working around the nail bed with circular movements.

2 With cuticle clippers very carefully snip away hang nails and loose skin.

3 After painting across the base of the nail, paint a strip of polish down the centre to the tip.

4 Fill in with a strip of colour on either side.

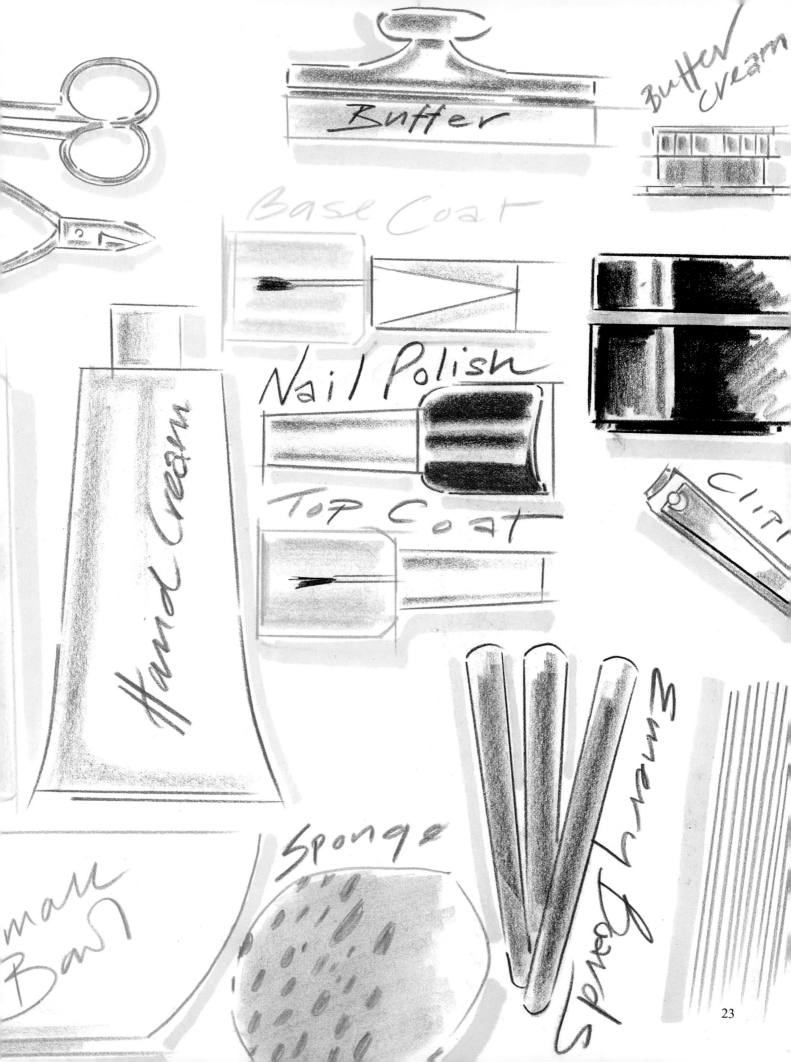

Buffer

Butter Cream

Base Coat

Nail Polish

Top Coat

Hand Cream

CUTI[...]

Sponge

Small Bowl

Emery Boards

Sponge Boards

23

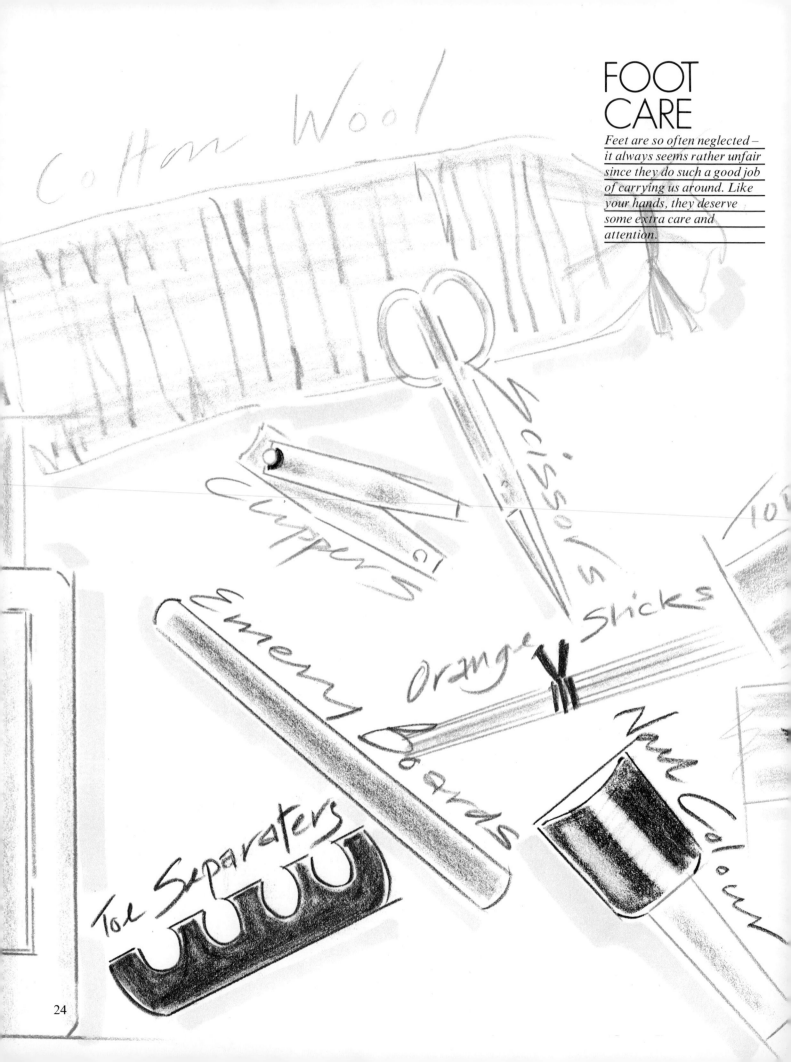

FOOT CARE

Feet are so often neglected – it always seems rather unfair since they do such a good job of carrying us around. Like your hands, they deserve some extra care and attention.

Cotton Wool

Scissors

Clippers

Orange Sticks

Emery Boards

Nail Colour

Toe Separaters

It goes without saying that badly fitting shoes won't do your feet any good, and it's a good idea to exercise regularly. Walking around indoors barefoot is one good exercise, or while you're sitting down try rotating each foot several times to the right, then several times to the left. Point your toes hard to extend your feet, then turn your toes upwards to flex them. Try picking small objects off the floor with your toes, and if you're standing still raise up on tip toes a couple of times.

If you have foot troubles such as bunions, corns, verrucae, or a heavy build-up of dry skin and calluses, you will need to consult a qualified chiropodist. Hacking away at one's own feet with scissors or razor blades is asking for trouble – it's easy to get an infection when skin is broken.

Otherwise to keep your feet looking nice and feeling smooth you can care for them with a pedicure, done in much the same way as a manicure for the hands. Even if feet are never considered attractive – they need never be ugly!

THE PEDICURE: applies to normal feet only. If your feet are abnormally dry or sweaty consult a qualified chiropodist. *First collect the things you will need . . .*
A bowl big enough for your feet, filled with warm water, and some soap
A towel
Nail scissors/clippers/nippers
Nail brush
Cotton wool
Emery board or nail file
Hand cream or body lotion
Nail polish – base coat and top coat if being used
Pumice stick or stone
Rubber 'toe separators' – or wrap a tissue round each toe to separate them

1 Rest and raise the feet for as long as you can.
2 Examine your feet for any specific problems such as verrucae, bunions, etc.
If you have no particular problems you can give yourself a simple pedicure.
3 Remove any old nail polish with an oily remover.
4 Trim the toe nails straight across, just slightly following the curve of the end of the toe.

Cut along the free edge only not down the sides.
5 Smooth off sharp corners with emery board or nail file.
6 Wash your feet in warm water for a few minutes. Use the nail brush to scrub your toe nails gently. Rub over dry or rough areas – for instance, the heel – with pumice, which will help smooth the dry skin. Dry each foot carefully, especially between the toes.
7 Massage your foot for a few minutes. Trim any hang nails that remain at the sides of your toes with cuticle clippers. Be super careful not to take off any more skin than is hanging free – and never cut all round the cuticle. It is especially important not to clip away the cuticle on your toe nail, since

toes need the cuticle to protect them from the pressures of shoes, and to avoid infection. You can neaten your cuticles by massaging a little baby oil into them once a week.
8 Apply hand or body lotion to your feet and legs. Work from the tips of your toes up to your ankles and on up to your knees.
9 Make sure no greasy cream is left on your toe nails if you intend to paint them.
10 Separate your toes with 'toe separators' or tissues. Apply a base coat, and top with nail polish. First paint a semi-circle of colour at the cuticle – leaving a hair's breadth between the polish and cuticle. Then paint the centre of the nail from base to tip. Fill in with two strokes down the sides.

EYEBROWS

Even if they're hidden under your fringe, eyebrows are vitally important to your looks. They can alter your face shape and change your whole expression. No matter what's fashionable – thin or thick – they should follow a natural line to suit your face shape.

Eyebrows are subject to changes of fashion, and so may be shaped in a way that's unsuitable for the face. All too often people pluck away too much hair from the brow, leaving a thin line that does nothing to balance the face shape. Whether the fashion is to wear eyebrows bushy or thin, one basic rule applies – you must have them beginning and ending in the right place. The beginning of an eyebrow is the beginning of the curve of your brow bone where it connects with the top of your nose. The eyebrow should be left to end where the hairs grow naturally, since most people's brow hair does not grow very far down past the outer corner of the eye.

To pluck your eyebrows you must clean your face really thoroughly – a good time to do it is directly after a bath when the skin is soft.

SHAPING YOUR BROWS

Collect together everything you'll need . . .

A good light
A mirror which is magnifying on one side if you are a little short sighted
Surgical spirit, or mild antiseptic lotion
Cotton wool
An eyebrow brush or comb, or old, clean toothbrush
A pair of tweezers – try to use tweezers which are small enough for you to handle easily, and have thin, flat, chisel-shaped tips

1 Tie hair well back from your face and position yourself in a good light – propping the mirror up so that you have both hands free.
2 Wipe the area lightly with the antiseptic solution.

3 Brush the eyebrows up into shape with the eyebrow brush and decide how much hair you wish to remove from the underneath. A good way to decide is to follow the natural shape of your eyebrow – leaving the lower edge a smooth, unbroken curved line by plucking away all the stray and unruly hairs.
4 Pull the hairs out by sliding the flat edge of the tweezer underneath a hair, gripping it firmly, and pulling sharply in the direction that the hair is growing. Continue this process until all superfluous hairs have been removed.

Some people find it helpful to pull the skin taut with two fingers of the other hand before pulling out the hair.

Cotton Wool

Anti septic

Headband

Toothbrush

Tweezers

5 Repeat the process on the other brow.

6 When you think you've finished plucking the hair from both eyebrows, brush them back into shape with the eyebrow brush and check – looking from one eye to the other – that they are in fact exactly the same.

7 Although it's not normally so necessary, if you have a lot of dark hairs growing above the brows and up to the hairline, you can pluck these areas too, as well as between your brows.

8 Wipe the area again with antiseptic lotion. And finally smooth on a little skin cream or moisturiser to help the now reddened area settle down. Don't make up your face until all the redness has gone and the skin is completely settled.

EYEBROW PROBLEMS

Overplucked Eyebrows

Sometimes it becomes impossible to grow back overplucked eyebrows, especially if the hair has been removed for long periods of time, because the hair follicles have been damaged for ever. However, if your eyebrows do grow back after being overplucked you may find they need a little help to encourage them to grow in the right direction. One of the best ways to do this is to comb or brush them as often as possible to make them lie flat. To help this process smooth a little vaseline on to them at night, and during the day if you're not wearing much eye make-up.

Straggly Brows

These can be treated in the same manner. If any of the brow hairs appear to be far too long or curly, either pull them out, or snip them shorter with nail scissors.

Pale or Blonde Eyebrows

If your eyebrows are far too fair for your general colouring you can tint them at home. One word of warning, however, if you use eyelash dye – remember it can look very heavy, so it's a good idea to apply it lightly. Take it off after

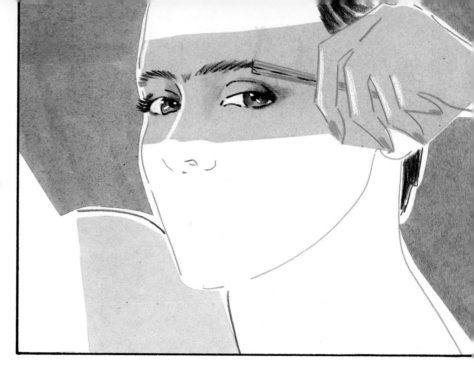

It is usually only necessary to pluck hairs from beneath the eyebrow. Slide the flat edge of the tweezer under the hair, grip firmly, and pull sharply in the direction that the hair is growing.

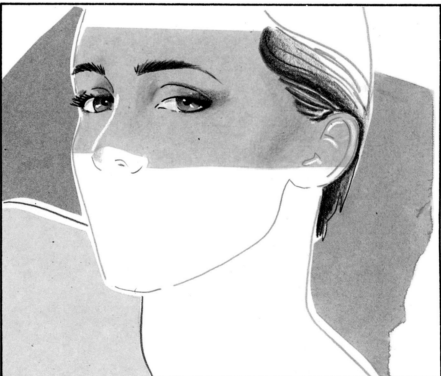

The perfect eyebrow follows the natural line of the brow in a smooth unbroken curve. It should start at the point where your brow bone connects with your nose, and finish naturally just above the outer corner of the eye.

a few minutes. If the brow isn't dark enough you can always repeat the process. Eyebrows, like eyelashes renew themselves about every 6 weeks so after a while the blonde hairs will start to grow through and you will have to repeat the process.

The easy alternative to dyeing your eyebrows is to etch them in with a soft brown or grey eyebrow pencil as part of your make-up routine. Draw a series of short feathery strokes rather than one hard unbroken line. Powder lightly, and brush into shape. Or, for a softer, more natural effect, brush brown powder eye shadow over your brows.

Most basic beauty treatments can be carried out at home and consistently good effects can be achieved with the minimum of equipment. There are, however, specialized treatments available in beauty salons that need the use of special equipment and expert therapists. Treatments for the body include saunas, steam cabinets, and massage equipment. Body massage given by a highly trained expert in a salon is indeed a very enjoyable and relaxing experience, and not something very easily done by amateurs.

If you happen to have

serious skin problems, such as severe acne, bad broken veins, or an extreme skin condition of some kind these will almost certainly be better treated by a highly trained beautician using a combination of beauty therapy and medical care, under the supervision of a doctor.

Although such treatments as leg waxing, etc., can be done by you, they're undoubtedly more efficiently, and perhaps more painlessly done by an expert, and certainly any form of electrolysis should never be attempted at home. Last, but of course, not least, most salons will do eyelash dyeing and make-up as well.

Brow brush

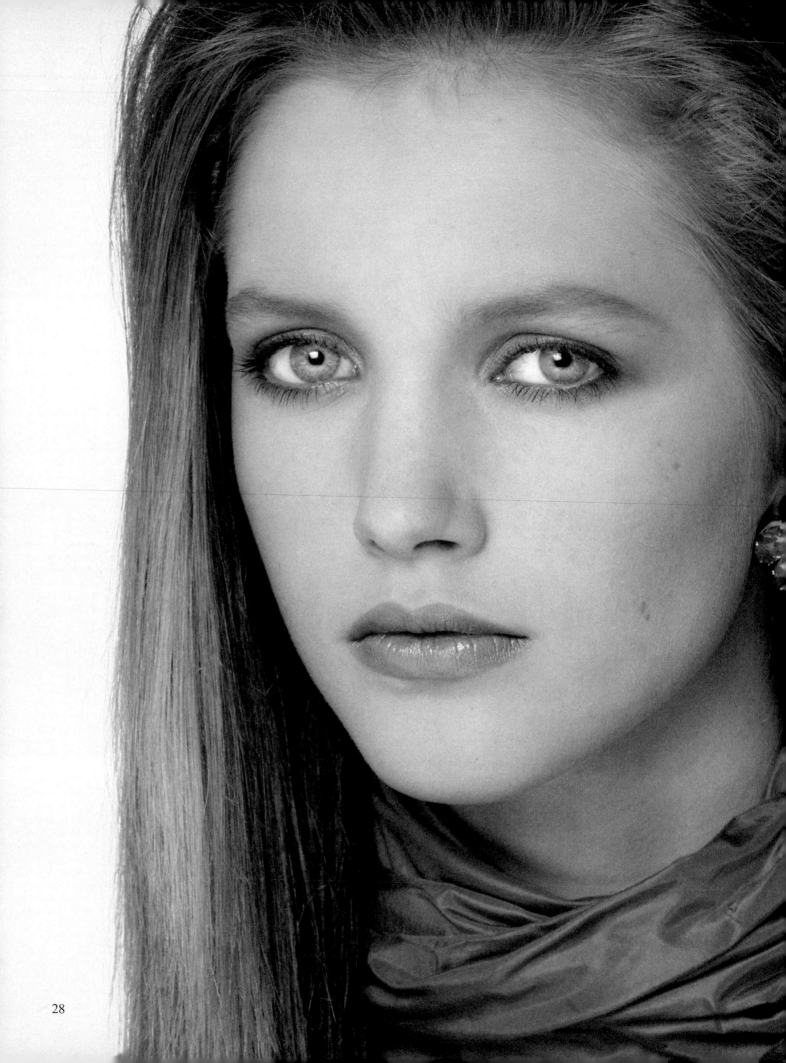

28

MAKE-UP

There is no such thing as a flawless face, but make-up can go a long way towards improving the face you have. It can make the very best of your potential, play up your good features so that no-one will ever notice the bad – and make you feel a whole lot better about your appearance.

Light is, without doubt, the single most important factor in making-up, in analysing your skin type and colour, and in buying and using your cosmetics. If you are to apply a make-up for day, and I mean the face you leave the house wearing each morning, you must put it on in the light it is going to be seen by. That is *daylight* – not a flattering soft bathroom light, or any old spot of light filtering through a small window, but 'full on-the-face daylight'.

At home, use natural light. Sit close to a window so that the light falls directly on to your face. Put your working equipment, table, dresser or whatever you are using in front of the light source. Light from either side won't do; side light throws shadows on to the unlit side of your face. If the room is darkish, or you're up early on a dark winter morning, or making-up for the evening, use lamps which you can point so that the light falls on to your face at eye level. I use two anglepoise lamps clipped to the top of a mirror. They should be as bright as possible, without dazzling you. In an emergency (someone else's house or a badly lit hotel room for instance) an ordinary table lamp, minus its shade, will do. But, remember, light can make or break your make-up.

FOUNDATION

Far from providing a heavy coverage, today's foundations are light and super subtle. They give a smooth finish and even skin tones – the basis of a perfect make-up.

The purpose of using a foundation on your skin is to make it look as naturally flawless as possible. It evens out skin tones and gives skin a smooth finish. What it *doesn't* do is change your skin colour, or leave your face looking heavily made-up. Not everyone needs to wear foundation, and if they do they may not need it over their whole face. For instance, if you have a generally good skin but you tend to have discolouration on your nose or chin, you may want to wear foundation just on these areas. Or if you have a young skin, or a much older, quite lined skin, you may need to use just a

Colour Corrective Cream

Concealers

Liquid Foundation

Foundation Cream

Sponge

Head band

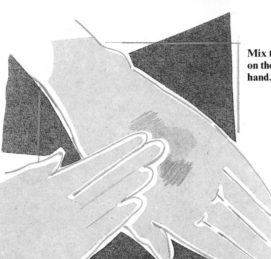

Mix the two colours
on the back of your
hand.

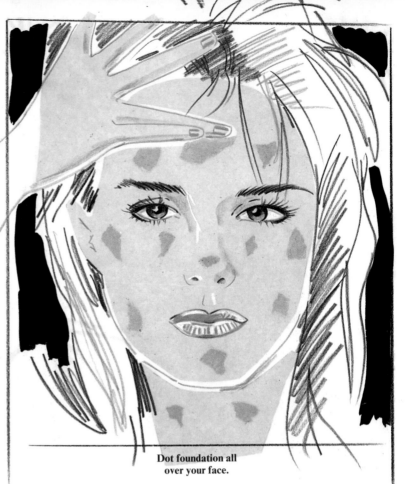

Dot foundation all
over your face.

little, thin foundation on the cheeks only, to even up the skin tones. The general rule is – use your foundation with discretion, and only as much as you need.

Buying Foundation
The type and colour of foundation you choose is determined by your own particular skin type. First decide how much coverage you feel you need.
Which Consistency? Heavy, thick foundations are really a thing of the past, now the lighter the better is the general rule. However, grease-based foundations are still available, mainly for stage work or very occasionally for heavy evening make-up.

Block foundations give the heaviest coverage of day-time foundations. You rub a damp sponge over them and apply directly on to your face.

Creams are still quite oily –

give medium coverage – and are good on dry skins. Avoid them on older skins, though, as they tend to settle in wrinkles.

Liquids are the most easily and widely used, and give a subtle, light coverage. They come in various thicknesses, and some contain added moisturisers. Others are water based and grease free for use on oily skins. They're often screened for skin irritants too, as are all foundations from hypo-allergenic cosmetic ranges, especially formulated for sensitive skins.

Which Colour? This is a difficult question for most people as there's an enormous range to choose from. Testing a foundation on your hand is not a good indication of how it will look on your face. You're looking for the shade that almost exactly matches your own complexion – not one that stands out. So pick two that you think are nearest and put a little of each on an un-made-up cheek. Take a look at them in *daylight*, using a hand mirror, and choose the one you're least aware of. If the colour you're looking for seems to be somewhere between the two, buy both. You can always mix them together yourself to achieve the colour you want.

Applying Foundation
Before you start, collect together the things you will need . . .
A good light source – in front of a window for day, or a lamp for evening
A mirror
Foundation
A damp sponge
A hairband, or clips to hold the hair back off your face

You will already have moisturised your skin. If you are mixing more than one foundation together, smooth a little of each on to the back of your hand and mix with a fingertip (see above).

Most foundations can be applied to the skin by dotting them on to the face (top right) and smoothing them in with a damp sponge, or with your fingertips (right). If using a sponge, do squeeze it out in a tissue first. If it is too wet it will just take your make-up off! Be careful not to push foundation too far into your hairline. Blend with the sponge just under the jawline, and fade away on to the neck.

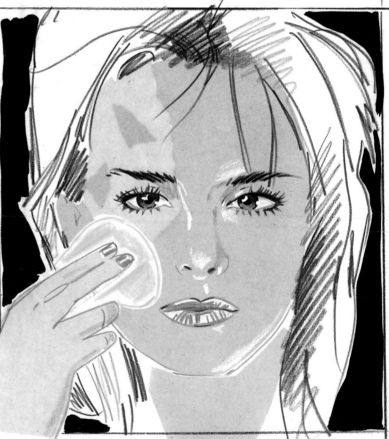

Blend with your
fingertips or a damp
sponge.

31

CONCEALERS, BLUSHERS, POWDER

To achieve a beautiful skin you also need a concealer to cover up blemishes, blusher to add colour, and face powder to refine the look of the skin and give it a smooth, matt texture.

Blusher Pencil

Face Powder

Concealers

Powders

Gel Blusher

CONCEALERS

After you have applied your foundation you may still have areas of darkness or discolouration under the eyes, around the nose, on the chin and cheeks; and the odd spot or pimple may still be visible. A heavier layer of foundation can just look darker – you need a concealer! Whether in a tube, pot or handy stick, concealers are, in fact, foundations with a very high content of pigment. That's what gives them their covering power. Some are medicated to help treat spots and pimples.

If your skin is one that doesn't normally need foundation all over, you may find that a concealer applied very lightly on the dark areas, i.e. under eyes, nose, etc., plus blusher and powder, may be all that you require to achieve a perfect looking skin.

Buying Concealer

Choose the colour that is nearest to your natural skin tone, in the same way as you would choose a foundation. Again, you may need to use more than one tone. They can be mixed in the same way as your foundation, or, indeed, with foundation.

Applying Concealer

Dot very tiny dots on the dark or discoloured areas, or over spots and pimples. Press or pat the concealer into the skin with your fingertips. Don't rub it, especially around the eyes.

BLUSHERS

Blushers are used to make the face look alive and the skin glow. They're *not* used for shaping the face, and one of the commonest mistakes is to draw a big wedge of red or pink down the sides of the cheeks in the hope that this will slim them. Careful placing of blusher can be used to flatter your face shape, but it's a subtle effect.

Blushers come as gels, liquids, creams, and powders, in tubes, sticks, bottles, pencils, jars, and compacts, but by far the most easy to use and therefore the most popular are the compressed powder compacts. These powders are always applied last, *after* your powder. All the others are liquid or cream based and go on *before* powder.

Buying Blusher

Don't be put off by the colour in the compact – often vibrant shades look a lot softer when they're blended into your skin, and you use only a tiny bit. It's a good idea to have at least two different shades, one bluey-pink and one peachy or tawny. That way you can match it up with the shade of lipstick you're wearing. The best idea is to try before you buy, if possible, but as a general rule choose a shade that will tone in with your skin colour – not stand out starkly. If your skin is slightly yellow buy peachy, orangey tones. If you're more pink, you need subtle roses and bluey pinks.

Applying Blusher

Apply powder blusher with the largest brush you have – the bristles of the brush spread the powder over your cheeks. Other kinds, liquids, gels, etc., can be applied direct with fingertips. Always blend the edges away very carefully so that there are no hard lines. Use a brush or sponge. Start with just a little blusher and build up if you need more. It's easier to add to your colour, than to take it away. Position the colour in the centre of your cheeks, but high up, away from the hairline, and not too close to the nose.

POWDER

Gone are the days when face powder was a thick heavy finish to make-up. Modern powder is light-weight, finely ground, and gives a perfect finish to the skin, as well as keeping the make-up underneath looking pristine all day. Powder is non-drying, so is fine for almost all skin types. Oily skin with open pores benefits particularly from its smoothing-out effect.

Powder can be bought in two forms – loose, which can be used direct from the container, or transferred to a compact; and compressed. A tiny amount of binding agent is used in compressed powder, so it may be slightly greasier than loose powder.

Buying Face Powder

You need the lightest, most transparent powder you can get. Remember you're not trying to colour your face with powder, just to lessen the shine slightly, and to 'set' the make-up underneath without changing its colours. Transparent powder isn't totally colourless, but it looks very pale in the box, and when brushed on to the skin almost disappears. Don't confuse the word translucent with transparent. Most modern face powder is called translucent – this just means that it has a good light-reflecting quality.

Applying Face Powder

It is not a good idea to use cotton wool – fibres can fly off and catch in eyelashes or go in your eyes. You're better off with a soft velour puff, or a large powder brush. Both are obtainable from cosmetic counters. And it's a good idea to have two of everything (either puffs or brushes) so that you can have one *clean* one ready for each new make-up.

Don't rub the powder on to your skin. Press it gently over your face, then brush off the excess lightly with puff or brush. If you rub you will remove the make-up underneath and cause streaking, so be very careful when 'setting' eye make-up.

It isn't always necessary to powder the entire face. Sometimes you need only powder shiny areas, such as nose, chin and forehead, and lightly over make-up on eyelids. People with older skins should certainly avoid excessive use of powder since it can 'settle' into fine lines.

Cream Blusher

Divine Stick

Powder Blusher

FACE SHAPES

SQUARE FACE

Make-up cannot change the shape of your face, but careful use of blusher and highlighter can have a subtle contouring effect. A square face can be given more curves by emphasizing the centre of the cheeks, and possibly highlighting the chin.

ROUND FACE

Round faces may look plump if blusher is in the wrong position. The right combination of blusher and highlighter helps to slim, lengthen and flatter the face.

LONG FACE

Long faces often have
attractive, well-defined
cheekbones. Make the most
of them with clever use of one
or two shades of blusher. A
dot of blusher on the tip of
the chin will help to shorten
it, but don't overdo it.

SQUARE FACE

Luckily, because of their very squareness, these have very well defined cheekbones.

Because square faces are also wide, it's a good idea to try and bring the cheek colour and emphasis well towards the centre of the face. This is done by keeping cheekbone highlight high to the sides of the face, and the blusher well forward on the cheek. Although square faces often have a prominent chin, some don't, and if you have a square face but need to make your chin look more pointed you can add highlight to the tip of it.

1 On our model concealer was applied as indicated within the dotted line – on dark shadows underneath the eye, and also near the bridge of the nose, to pull the eyes apart.
2 Highlighter was applied to the cheekbone and chin and blended well with fingertips and a cosmetic sponge.
3 The blusher, which in this case was a pencil, and therefore applied before the face powder but on top of the foundation, was blended carefully with a damp cosmetic sponge. The edges were faded away towards the outside of the face, while the strongest depth of colour was kept well to the centre of the cheek.

Tip For Evening
After you have finished your eye make-up, brush a little blusher across the outer edges of the browbone as well as on the temples. Add a small dot of highlighter to the centre of your browbone to give the eyes extra sparkle.

ROUND FACE

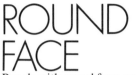

People with round faces usually have smaller noses and often full lips.

Although make-up can't change the shape of the face, it is important to remember that where you put your blusher and highlighter will either emphasise the roundness of your face, or help to give it a little more contour.

After applying foundation, use concealer to cover dark shadows and to highlight any areas you wish to emphasise. Then use face powder if you're going to use a powder blush, or apply a cream blusher first and follow with powder.

1 On our model under-eye shadows were concealed as shown with dotted lines.
2 A little concealer mixed with an off-white face highlighter cream was used to emphasise the cheekbones and the chin. Be careful to blend these very carefully so they don't look like white patches on your face. Do use your make-up sponge to help you blend.
3 The face was powdered.
4 Powder blush was applied in a downward shape as indicated within the area of the dotted line. The blush was smoothed carefully into the skin so that there were no hard edges. When you're using a powder blush remember to use a nice fat blusher brush, one especially made for the job that will help you blend the colour evenly over your cheeks.

Tip For Evening
When highlighting your face emphasise the cheek highlight by brushing on a shiny powder. Add a little of the same shiny powder to the tip of your chin, and put a touch lightly down the centre of your nose.

LONG FACE

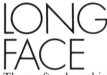

These often have high cheekbones and slender noses. Without trying to alter your face shape you will find the correct placing of your blusher, or blushers if you decide to use more than one colour, can help you make the face look shorter and emphasise the naturally high cheekbones.

The first step is to apply your foundation if you are wearing one. The second is to use your concealer to cover any dark shadows or blemishes, and the third is to apply your blushers. Remember the rule of cream or pencil blusher *under* face powder; powder blushers *over*.

1 On our model the dark shadow under the eye has been disguised with concealer, applied to the area within the dotted line, and blended by patting and pressing gently into the skin.
2 The cheek blush was applied across the cheek as indicated, and blended gently, especially at the edges. A cream blusher was used, which was blended with the fingertips, and finally smoothed over with a damp cosmetic sponge.

The slightly darker blush was applied below this to give some extra moulding to the cheek, and was blended into the blusher above. Translucent powder gave the finishing touch and set the blusher.
3 A small dot of blush was well blended into the tip of the chin to help shorten it. Be very careful if you do this not to end up with a pink chin.

Tip For Evening
Put an extra glow on your skin by very lightly fluffing a little of your blusher on to your temples as well as on your chin.

From subtle shades, to startlingly bright colours – eye make-up today can be anything you want it to be. Your eyes are the focus of your face. And with the fantastic range of colour combinations to choose from, who could resist experimenting?

EYES

Buying Eye Make-Up
The Basic Needs There are two main types of eye shadow – grease based, and powder based. Although gels are sometimes used, particularly in summer. Grease-based shadows include creams in sticks, pots, wands and tubes, as well as pencils of all kinds, such as eyebrow pencils, and powder-cream pencils. Creams crease easily, and are more messy, less controllable to use than powders. Pencils are very easy to apply just where you want them, and handy for carrying around.

Powders are quick and easy to apply, and long lasting. They're usually available in compacts and palettes.

For a good eye make-up you'll also need eyeliner – either pencil, liquid, or block, which you wet with water and apply with a brush; and mascara – in a wand or block.

Kohl is a black powder traditionally used to line the *inner* rim of the eye. Nowadays, soft dark-coloured eye pencils in black, brown or navy blue, have been specially formulated to replace the powder for easier use. You can in fact use most eye pencils inside the eye, but check the printing on the package first for warnings against this.
Glitter and Shine Almost all types of eye shadow can be bought with some kind of shine, pearl, or even glitter in them. Again, the range of colours is enormous. Very pale, shiny shadows, such as cream, pale pink or blue, are used to highlight the eye, and can look pretty for day-time make-up. Other, more highly pearlised or metallic, glittering eye shadows look ludicrously hard in daylight and are best kept for

evenings. Pearly eye shadows emphasise crêpiness, and can irritate sensitive eyes – so if you have an older skin, or are prone to allergies, avoid shiny shadows.

Applying Eye Make-Up
Best Equipment Good brushes are the key to a good eye make-up, along with the right light (see page 29), and a mirror – magnifying, if you're a little short sighted. Most eye make-up comes with some kind of applicator these days, and packs of extra applicators can be bought, but a soft brush, about $\frac{1}{4}$ inch wide, will usually give you a better, more controlled finish. If you want to obtain a really professional look invest in two or three good artists' brushes. Look for the ones that have 'chisel' ends. Most good art shops have them. Be careful never to wash real hair brushes – clean them with a little dry-cleaning fluid (carbon tetrachloride). Wipe the CTC off with a tissue, and make sure it has had time to evaporate away before you use the brush again. This way your equipment will last for years.

Cotton buds are good for cleaning up the odd mistake, and should be used damp. An eyelash brush or comb is essential for brushing out eyebrows, and separating lashes after applying mascara. You can keep an old, clean toothbrush for eyebrows, if you like. If you're using block mascara and eyeliner, always have an egg cup full of clean water ready to wet them.

The Basic Rule of Eye Make-Up
Remember, use all *grease-based* eye make-up, i.e. cream eye shadows, pencils, eyebrow pencils, etc., *after* foundation but *before* you powder your face. They have to be set with the face powder, otherwise they will crease quickly on the eye.

All *powder-based* eye make-up – compact shadows, or pots of powder, should be applied *after* powdering the face.

Eyeliner and mascara are

always done last, *after* face powder and eye shadow.

EYE SHAPES
Eyes can be divided into two basic categories of 'shape' depending on the size of the lid.

The first is the deep-set or 'small' eye, where there isn't much lid showing. This kind of eye often has a narrow area between the line of the upper lashes and the eyebrow, and no well defined socket.

The second is the 'protruding' eye, which has a rather prominent upper lid.

Apart from these differences, eyes are all more or less the same almond shape, set in different shaped sockets.

Therefore, when considering what to do with your own eye make-up you need only assess how much lid you have to work with. If there isn't a lot of lid showing, keep darker eye shadows towards the outer edge of the eye, and lighter colours from the centre of the eye inwards, towards the nose.

If you think your eyes look too full or protruding, keep the colour stronger at the centre of the lid, and gradually fade it away to the outer and inner corners of the eye. Keep shadows soft and matt on protruding eyes or on very full eyelids – shiny eye shadows will only emphasise the problem. *Remember:* Dark, matt colours recede problem areas; light shiny colours emphasise your good points.

Brushes

Aplicator

Wand

Egg cup

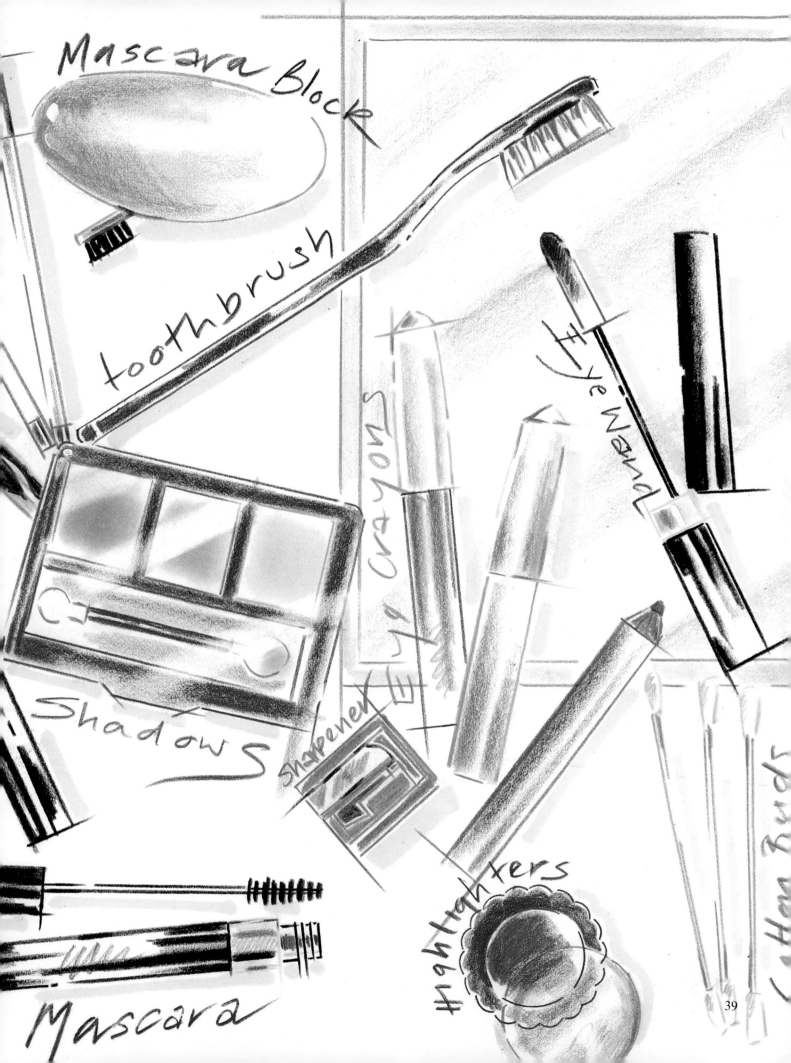

Mascara Block

toothbrush

Eye Wand

Eye Crayons

Shadows

Sharpener

Highlighters

Mascara

Cotton Buds

39

BLUE EYES

Of course if you want to you can always wear blue eye shadow with blue eyes. When the colour match is perfect this sometimes enhances their colour, but mostly blue on blue deadens the natural colour of the eye and looks very hard. Blue eyes often look bluer with a contrasting eye shadow. Good colours are golden brown, slate grey, rose pink, copper and khaki. In this make-up I've combined peach, rust, and copper shadows with a slate blue mascara to give extra impact.

40

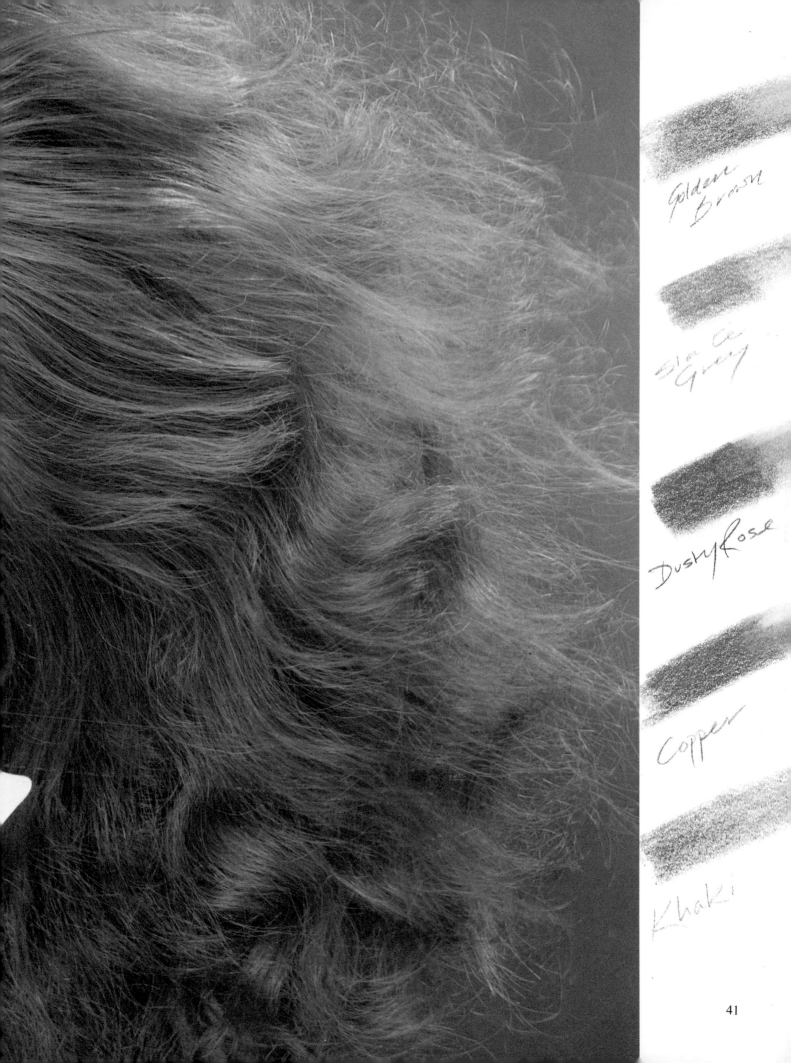

Golden Brown

Slate Grey

Dusty Rose

Copper

Khaki

41

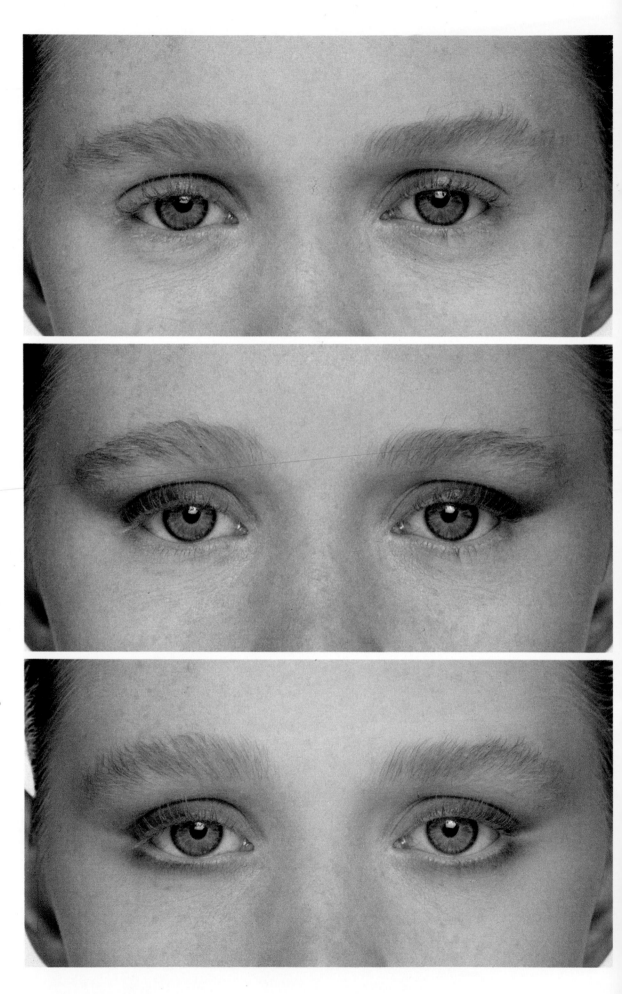

1 On upper eyelid, fill in from the inner corner to the centre of the lid with a peach pencil eye shadow. Blend upwards towards the eyebrow.

2 Emphasise upper lash line with a line of rust-coloured pencil, blended outwards and upwards.

3 Add a copper pencil line beneath the lower lashes, and blend slightly with a brush to soften.

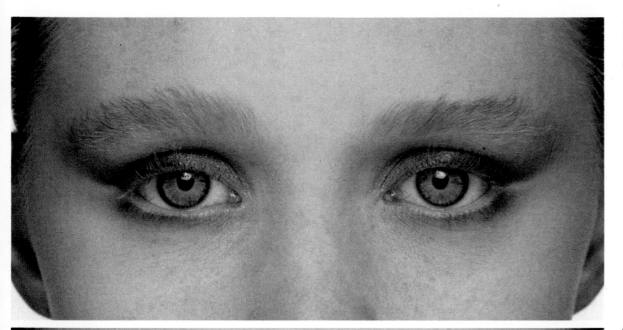

4 Highlight the inner half of the upper eyelid with a shiny copper eye shadow.

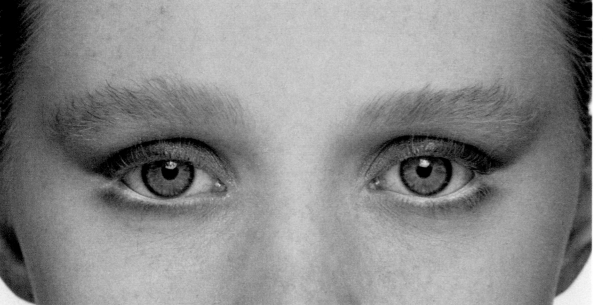

5 Apply white kohl pencil to the inside of the lower lash rim, and a touch of white at the outer corners of the eyes. This makes the eyes look wide open.

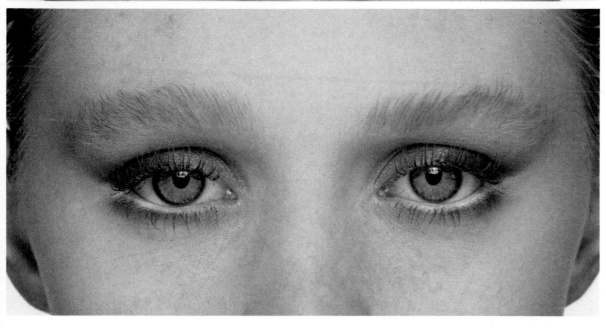

6 Finish with slate blue mascara on the eyelashes. Use an eyelash comb to separate the lashes, making sure none are left sticking together.

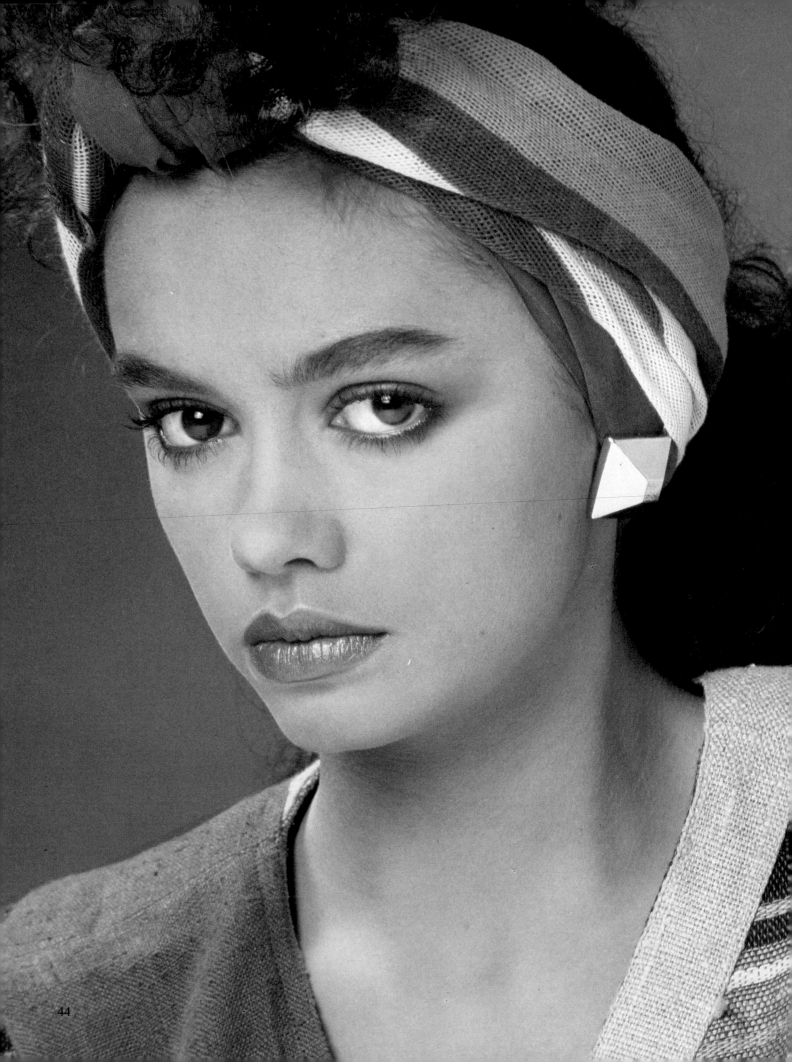

BROWN EYES

These can be accompanied by dark or light hair and skin, so when choosing your eye make-up take your natural colouring into consideration. If you have very dark colouring, deep eye colours can make your eyes look too heavy. But you can get away with using dark shadows if you add a lighter colour for contrast. Good colours for brown eyes are dark brown, violet, gold, coral and bottle green. In this make-up a touch of brown shadow defines the eye shape, but violet and gold are the major, lighter colours.

Dark Brown

Violet

Gold

Coral

Bottle Green

45

1 Follow the shape of the socket line with a lavender pencil eye shadow. Blend with a brush towards the eyebrow.

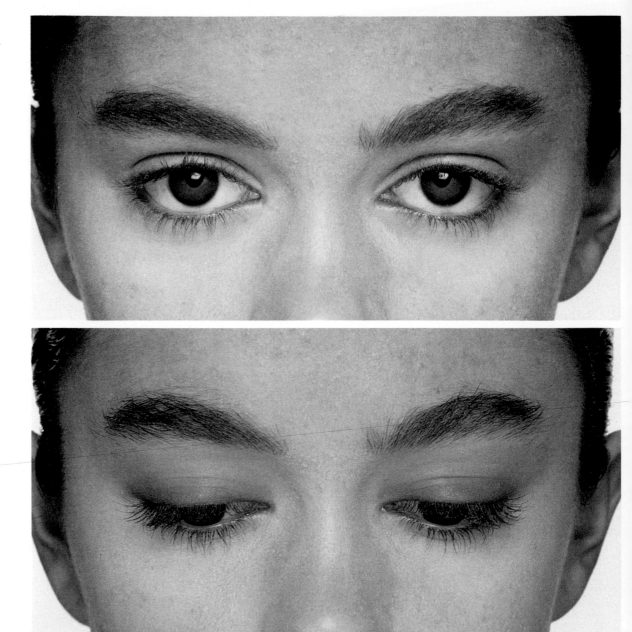

2 Blend violet eye shadow right across the upper lid.

3 Powder the eyes with transparent powder to set the pencils.

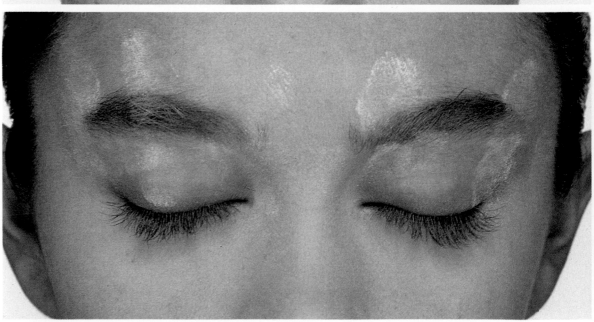

46

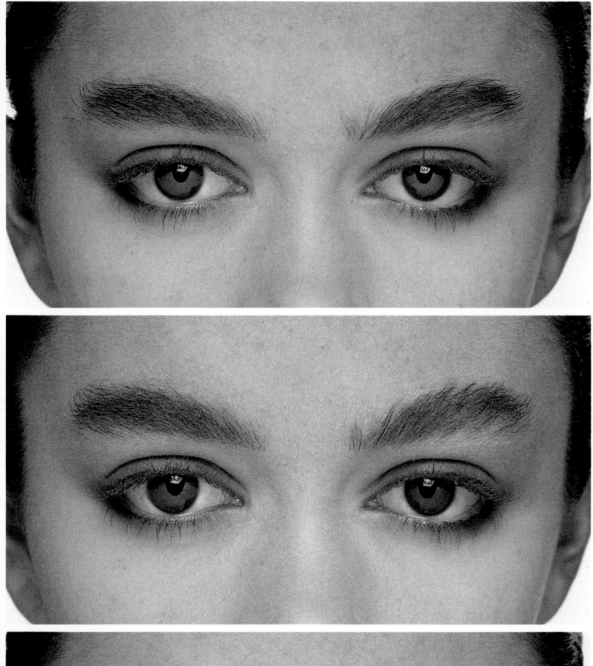

4 Define the lower outer corners of the eyes with a small amount of dark brown powder eye shadow.

5 Highlight the browbone with gold powder eye shadow, and smooth it slightly up over the temples.

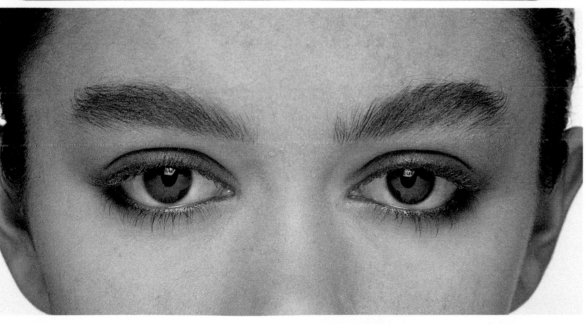

6 Draw a line of bluey-violet kohl pencil inside the rim of the lower lashes, and add black mascara.

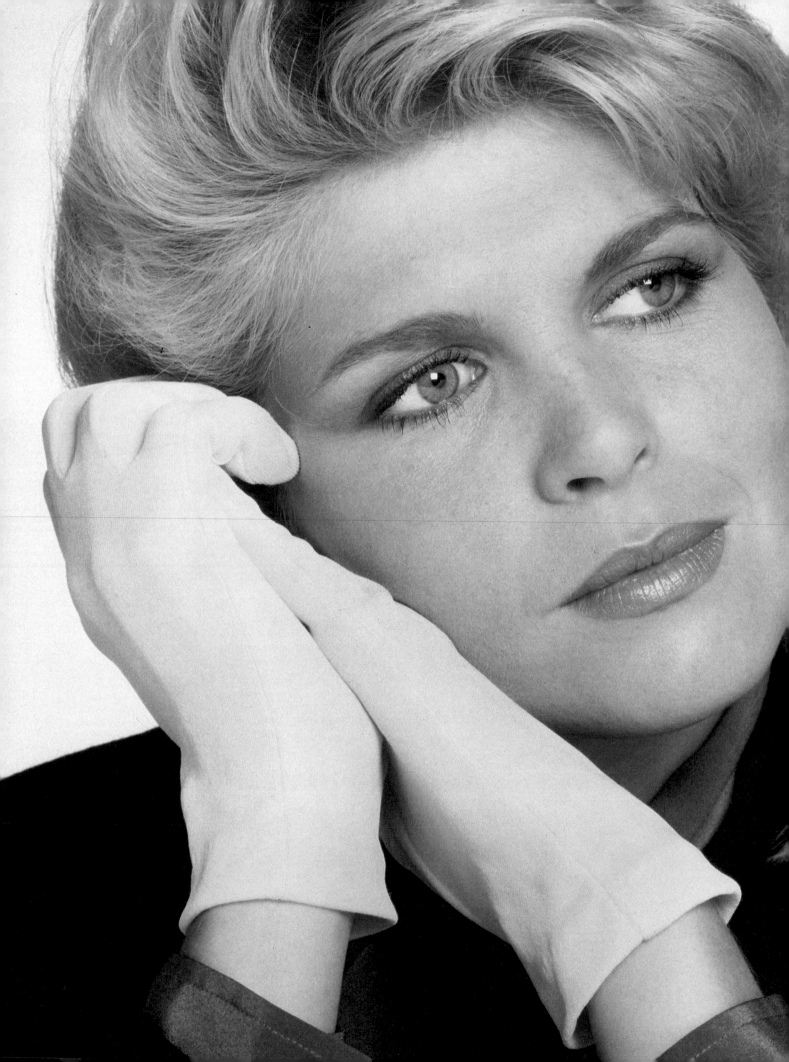

GREEN EYES

These are quite unusual, and can vary in shade from blue-green to bright green to hazel, a mixture of brown and green, and can often have tones of yellow or aquamarine. Look closely at your eyes to see what colours they're composed of. You can choose a contrasting colour – or one that matches the shade of your eyes. Good contrasting colours to wear with green eyes are yellow, green-grey, blue, apricot and mid-brown. In this make-up I've used yellow-green rather than blue-green shadow – it's better for hazel eyes. A touch of brown complements the flecks of gold in the eyes.

Yellow

Green Grey

Blue

Apricot

Mid Brown

1 Cover your entire upper lid with a peach pencil eye shadow.

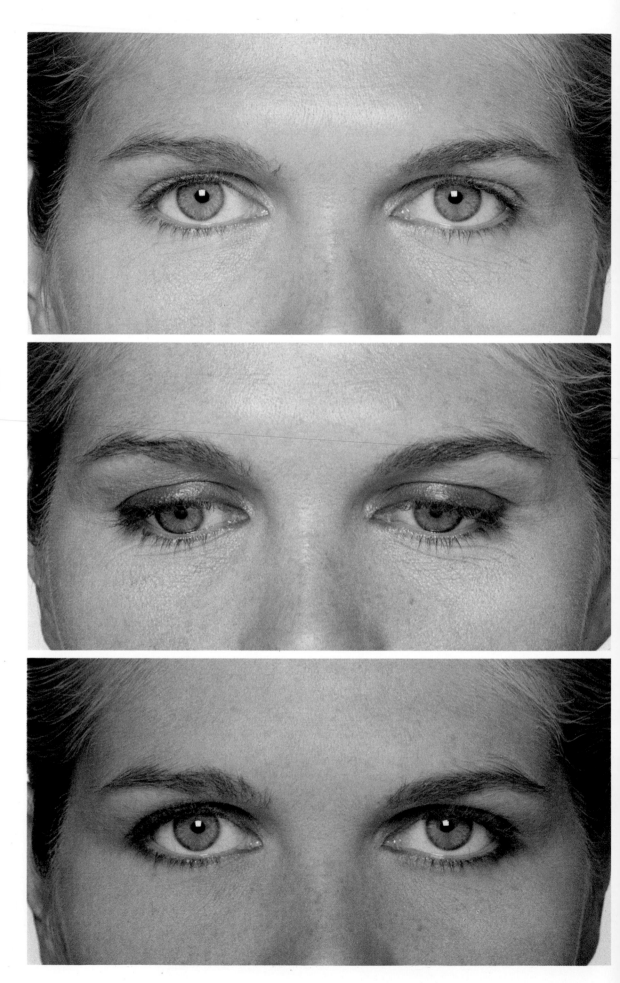

2 Emphasise the eye shape with a brown pencil line along upper lashes. Blend to soften with a brush, and powder lightly with transparent powder.

3 Define under the lower lashes with a little blended forest green powder shadow.

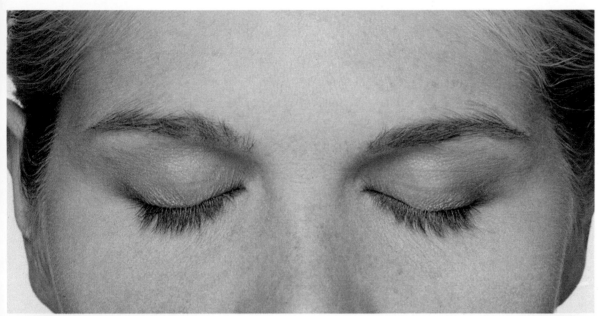

4 Highlight the centre of the upper lid with a yellow powder shadow.

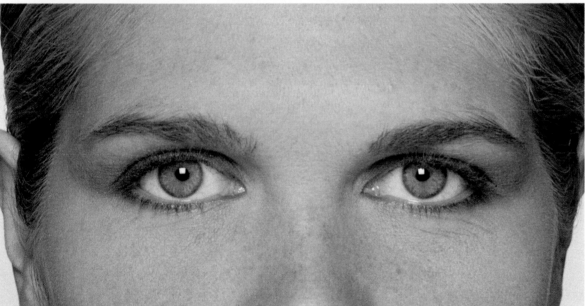

5 Brush apricot eye shadow into the socket line and blend away towards the eyebrows.

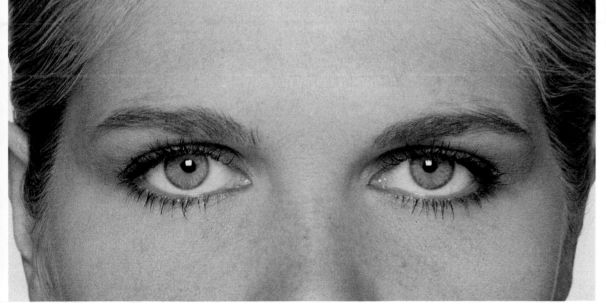

6 Apply black mascara to eyelashes. Emphasise the eye shape with a fine line of light green kohl pencil on inner rim of eye. Comb eyelashes.

GREY EYES

These often appear to change colour according to what you are wearing. For instance, grey or blue-grey eye shadows will emphasise their greyness, whereas a colour contrast will make them look either bluer or enhance the natural lightness of the grey. Grey eyes are often accompanied by light skin and hair and therefore don't look good surrounded by very bright or very dark colours. Good colours for grey eyes are air force blue, navy, silver, ochre, emerald green and a clear pink. In this make-up silver and grey team perfectly with navy for beautifully bold eyes.

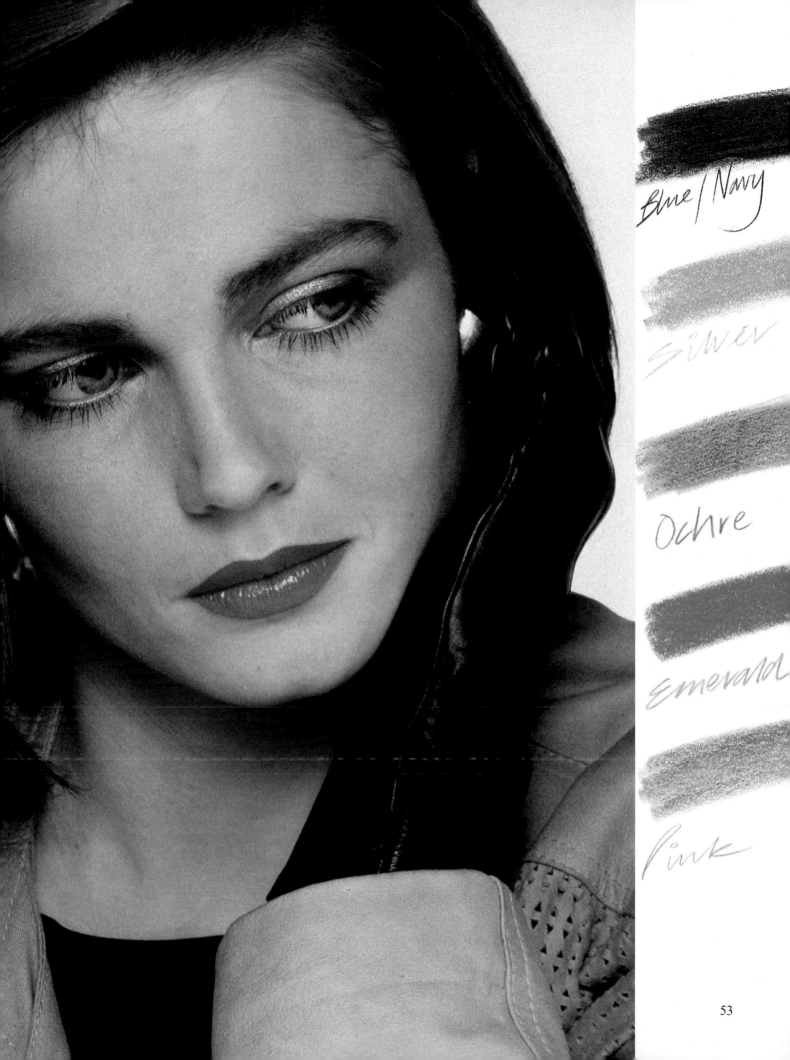

Blue/Navy

Silver

Ochre

Emerald

Pink

53

1 Blend a pale silvery-grey eye shadow over the whole lid, and fade it away up to the brow.

2 Outline the outer rim of the upper lid and outer edge of lower lid with a navy blue eye pencil.

3 Elongate the eye shape by applying a navy blue powder eye shadow to the outer half of the upper lid.

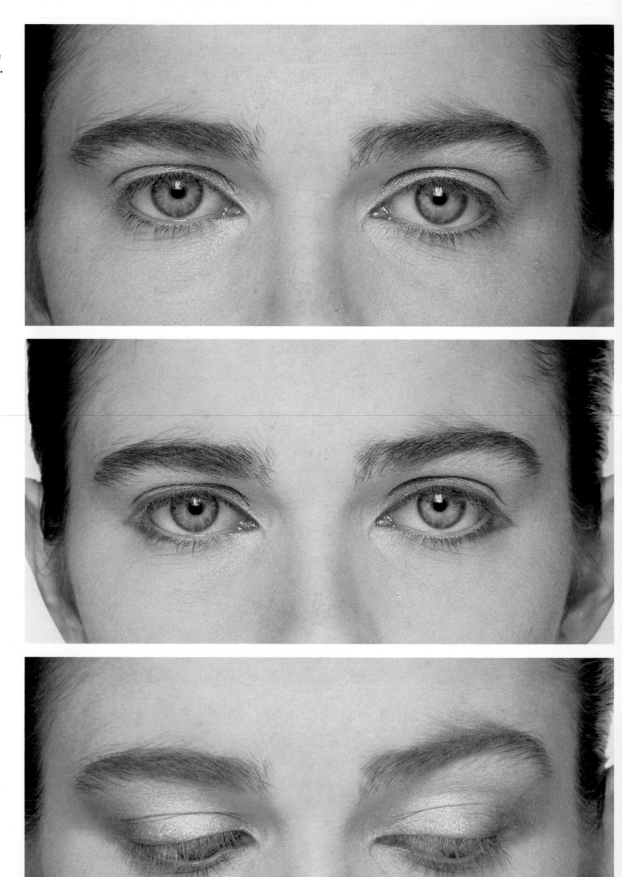

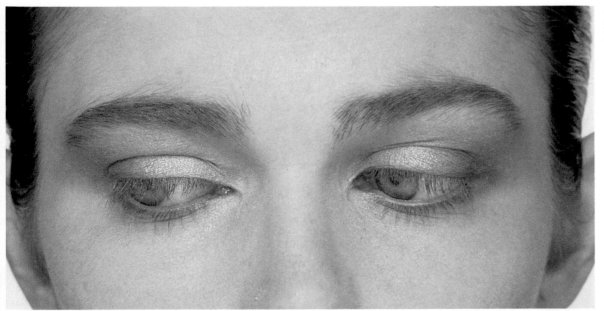

4 Blend pink eye shadow into the socket line, and slightly down over the lid.

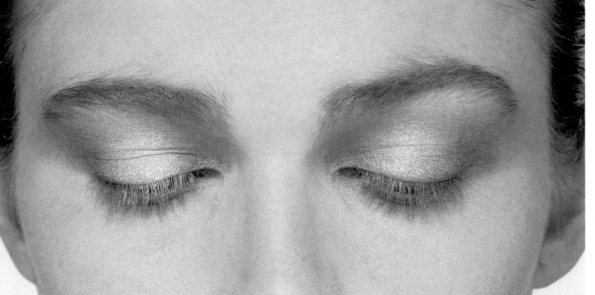

5 Brush a very soft grey eye shadow into the inner corners of the eyelid.

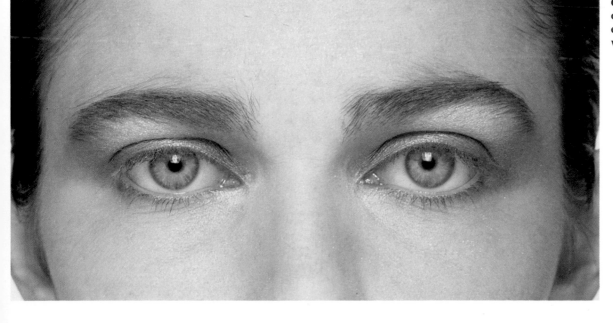

6 Highlight the centre of the lid with silver eye shadow, and finish with black mascara.

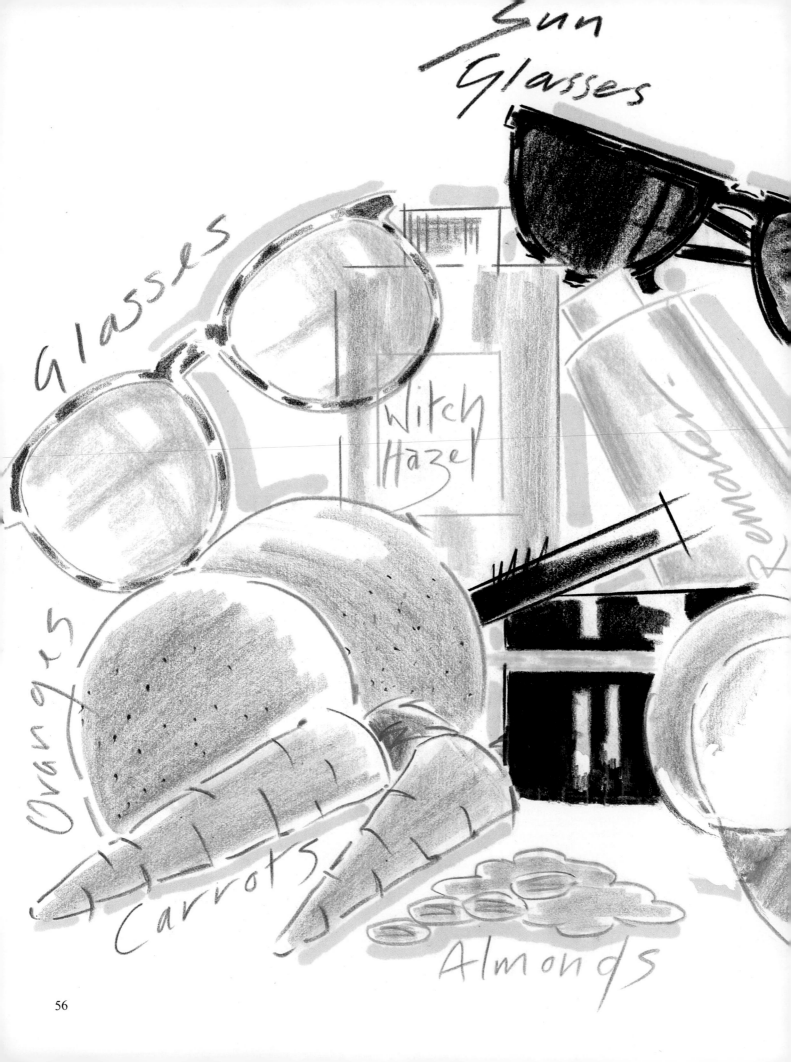

Sun
Glasses

Glasses

Witch
Hazel

Oranges

Carrots

Almonds

56

EYE CARE

Healthy eyes are beautiful eyes – no matter what their shape and colour. Your eyes mirror the health of your whole body and also reflect the state of your mind.

If you are under stress, worried and overtired it shows in your eyes. It is often the first place that a doctor inspects when you visit him. So the old saying that the eyes are indeed the mirrors of your soul, seems to be true.

The Importance of Diet

To keep your eyes healthy one of the first golden rules is to have a well balanced diet containing the right kinds of vitamins for your eyes. The foods which contain ample amounts of Vitamin A – the most important vitamin for eye health – are yellow vegetables and fruit; carrots, oranges and swedes, for example. Nuts, such as almonds, also contain large amounts of Vitamin A. It's not necessary to eat vast amounts of these foods but they should be part of your everyday diet.

Eye Exercises

Your eyes need exercise just as much as the rest of your body. If we were living in a totally natural environment we would exercise our eyes by constantly altering our focus from far distances to objects close at hand. While working eight hours at home or in an office, we tend to focus our eyes at objects that are no more distant than the length of our living room or office desk. It's a good idea to spend a minute or two every now and again during your day looking at something far away and then quickly focusing on something very near. Repeat this a few times to exercise the muscles. Look around you, circling the eyes in each direction several times, to complete the exercise.

Check-Ups

If you suffer from any form of eye strain check that you always work or read using a really good light source, and if the strain seems to persist, don't hesitate to have your eyes checked in case you need glasses. It's a good idea to have your eyes checked every few years anyway, because eyes change as you grow older. Your vision may have been perfect at seventeen, but at twenty-seven it may need a little help. If you find yourself squinting either at distances or close up, you can be pretty sure that you need to have your eyes tested. Most opticians carry a marvellous range of glasses these days, so there's something to suit everyone. The right glasses worn when needed are a lot more attractive than frown lines and crows' feet caused by squinting.

Removing Make-Up

Everyone can wear eye make-up these days – even people with very sensitive eyes can find products in hypo-allergenic ranges which will flatter and enhance them, without causing irritation. But if you're going to wear make-up, it's very important that you remove it properly at the end of the day.

We all know people who claim they never remove their mascara, and have never had an infection – but it isn't a good idea. You do run the risk of infection if you allow bacteria to cling to the base of your lashes, and stay there, lodged in old eye make-up for days on end. To remove eye make-up thoroughly you need a cleansing agent specially designed for the job – liquids or oils in bottles, creams in tubes, or eye make-up remover pads impregnated with oil. Try them out to find the one you like best. Oily removers work fastest, but can leave a film over your eyes.

Whichever you choose, never rub your eyes when removing make-up. They are suspended in their sockets and the skin around them is not supported by strong muscle – pulling it will make it sag. When using your remover you can either massage it gently over your eyes with your fingertips, and then remove with damp cotton wool, or you can apply it directly on damp cotton wool, and remove it with more. Don't drag the eyes with a tissue – and if little bits of make-up really cling to the base of the lashes, dip a cotton bud in remover and use it to lift the make-up.

Protection

Sleep, of course, is an important factor in eye health, as well as in our general well-being. If you don't get enough of it, or even if you sleep too much, your eyes can look red rimmed and puffy. One way to reduce this puffiness is to lie down with some eye pads over your eyes, impregnated with eye lotion. You can buy them, or make your own by soaking two pads of lint in eyebath solution or witch hazel. If you really don't have either, two cold teabags are quite soothing.

Last, but not least, remember to take care of your eyes at all times. Don't abuse them by sitting in strong sunlight, or using sun beds or lamps without protection from glasses or goggles. Remember that your eyes are not replaceable.

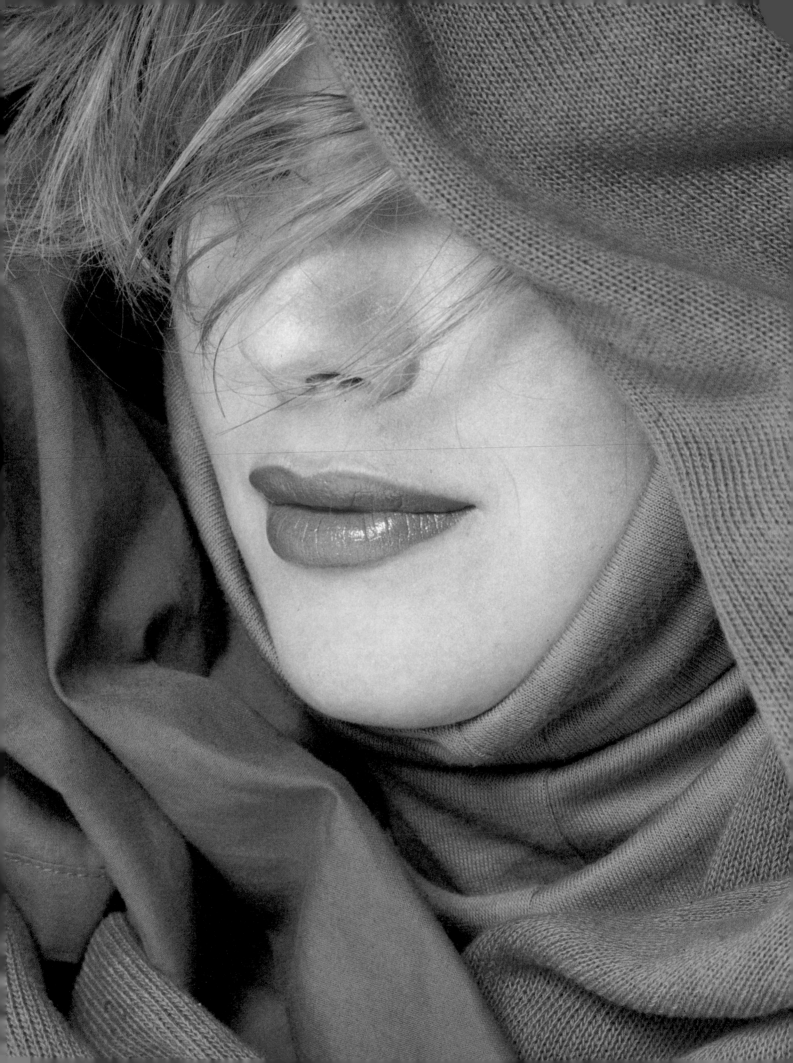

LIPS

Shocking red, or palest pink – the colour of your lips says a lot about you. Your lips are the sexiest part of your face. Whether you play them up, or keep them subtle, they should look soft and shapely – and that's where lipstick comes in!

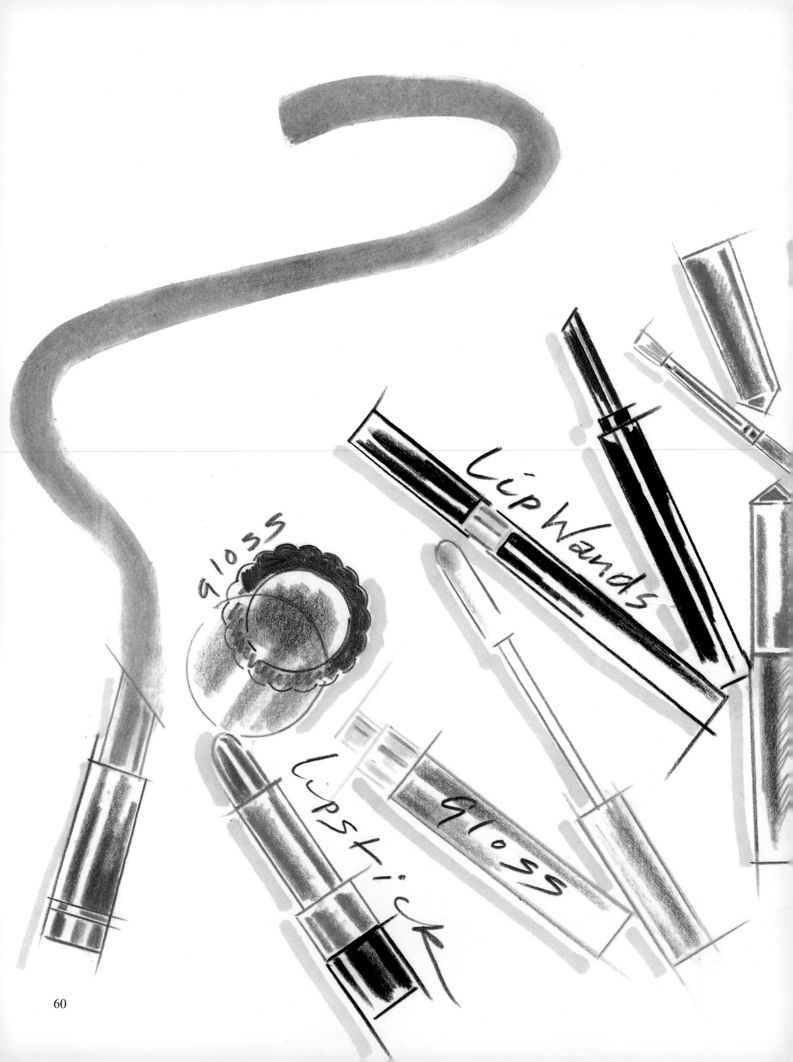

gloss

Lip Wands

gloss

Lipstick

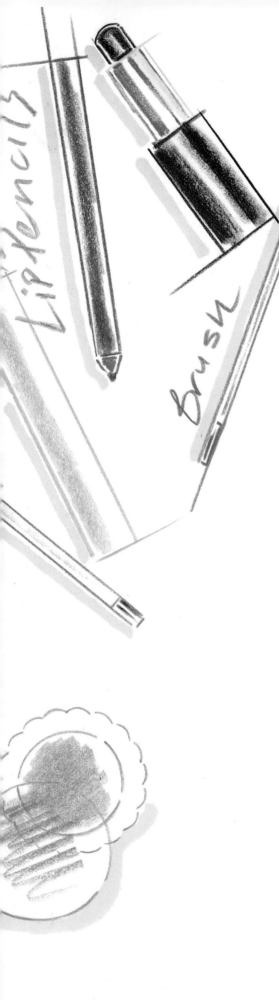

Lip Pencil(s)

Brush

LIP COLOURS

Lip make-up of some kind seems always to have been used by women, and sometimes by men, in most countries of the world.

Although lips sometimes appear in dark blue, yellow or other 'unnatural' colours we mostly choose to echo nature's original tone, and therefore lipsticks come in every conceivable shade of red, ranging from the palest of violet pinks to the deepest of burgundies. Lip colour can add a whole new dimension to your face. The colour you choose can emphasise or detract from the natural shape of your mouth, and complement the colour of your skin, hair, and eyes. It is one of the most useful fashion accessories and can be used to pick up a colour in your clothing to very good effect.

Lipsticks come in many forms – regular lipstick, with which we're all familiar; colour in compacts, usually supplied with their own brush; colour in pots; lipstick in wands and lipstick in pencils. There are also thinner pencils of a harder formula to outline the lips.

The kind of product you use is entirely up to you. Some people get along very well with lipstick in a wand form, used in conjunction with a lip liner pencil, others prefer tube lipstick. Everyone needs a wardrobe of lip colours. It doesn't need to be vast, although we all tend to collect lipsticks more than any other type of cosmetic.

A good basic colour collection would be a soft browny pink; a copper colour; a red or as near red as you feel you can comfortably wear; and a bright pink, which can look wonderful worn at full strength or can be used sparingly just to enliven the face. If you wear a lot of warm colours in your clothing it's a good idea to have a peachy, orange lip colour to wear with them.

You don't need to be overly concerned by whether or not your lip colour is 'good' for your hair or eyes. Most people can wear most colours and most people know what colours suit them, for instance if you are the sort of person who never wears navy blue, you can be sure that lipsticks with dark bluish overtones won't suit you. So let your own colour sense be your guide.

Do be adventurous though – it's amazing what a change of lip colour can do for your whole appearance. You may feel you couldn't possibly wear a red lipstick – and yet if you wear red clothes or accessories you'd probably do very well wearing red lip colour in a softer tone.

LIP SHAPES

Although you can, to some extent, give the impression of making your mouth larger or smaller by using your lipstick in a certain manner, it isn't a good idea to try to overpaint or underpaint more than a hair's breadth on either side of your natural lip line.

If you do want to alter your lip shape you must learn to draw a clean outline using either a lip brush or a lip liner pencil. Remember that darker lip colours will tend to make your mouth look smaller, although they will also draw attention to it, and that lighter lip colours can make the mouth look fuller. If you want to wear a dark or bright lip colour, but also want to make your mouth look fuller, you can use a highlight – for instance a pearly lip gloss – in the centre of the bottom lip.

Using a lip pencil or a lip brush will help to prevent lipstick bleeding. Lip treatment creams are also available now, which when applied before a lip colour will help to stop it running. Blotting your lipstick well and lightly powdering the edges of the line before you add more lipstick or gloss to the centre of the mouth is another safeguard against spidery runs.

Finally, of course, you need to keep the skin of your lips smooth. A sun protector is vital in hot weather to stop burns and cracking, as is the liberal use of a lubricant and protector, such as vaseline or an anti-chap stick, in the cold of the winter.

1 If you want a fairly natural look, but your lips do need some definition, use a brownish pink pencil to outline them. Make sure the pencil has a sharp point so that the outline will be clear-edged and crisp.

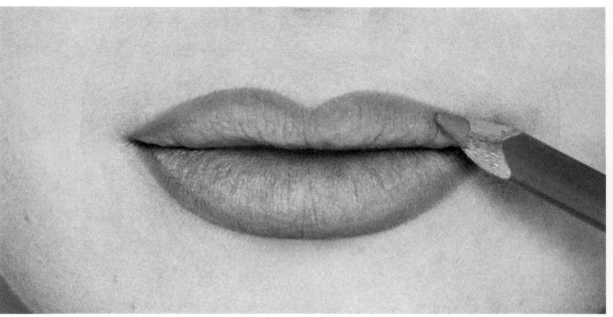

Fill in with a matching lipstick colour, blot lightly and top with a very thin coat of lip gloss for a finished effect that is soft and natural looking.

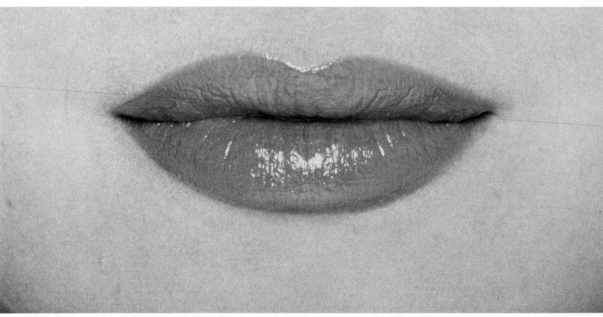

2 A clean crisp outline is especially important when using darker shades of lipstick. A good edge will improve the shape of your lips, and help your lipstick last longer. In this case I used a chisel-shaped lip brush, but you could choose a pencil if you prefer. When using a brush, always smooth any excess lipstick on to the back of your hand first.

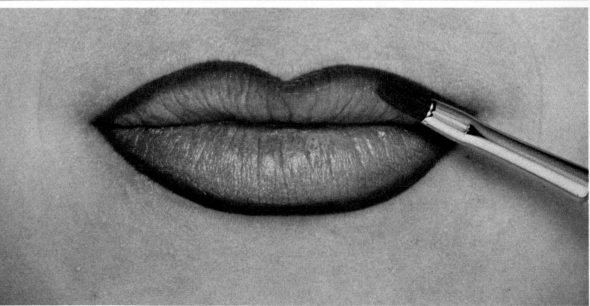

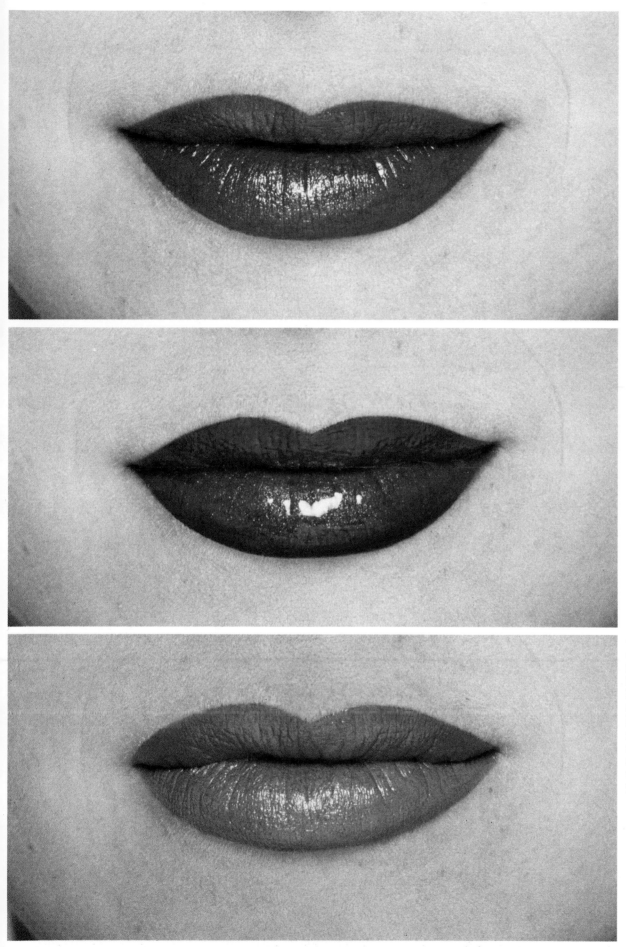

Fill in with a toning colour and then blot your lips. If you want to stop the edges running, powder very lightly, and brush on a little more lip colour if you like.

3 Make a vivid lip colour look softer by applying the colour all over the lips, and then highlighting the centre bottom lip with a gold or silver lip gloss. This is a very special look for evening.

4 A particularly effective way of making the lips look a little fuller is to use a lighter shade of the same tone on the bottom lip. Be careful not to choose a colour that is *too* light since it could look odd against the darker tone on your upper lip.

LOOKS FOR LIFESTYLES

DIFFICULT COLOURS

Whatever fashion dictates as the seasonal colours for our clothes, there's always a way to co-ordinate your make-up. At first sight the colours may seem hard to wear and difficult to match with make-up. But though you may not be able to wear all the colours on your face, you can pick out the strongest colour and match or tone an eye colour to it. If it happens to be a non-eye-make-up colour, red, for instance, keep your eyes fairly neutral, and choose a lipstick to match.

An ivory-toned foundation was applied to our model's face to even out skin tones. Pale yellow cream eye shadow was smoothed over the whole eyelid and blended away up to the brow. This provided a base on which to add more colour. Next, the socket line was defined with a line of khaki-green eye pencil, which was blended to soften. Grey pencil gave definition to the outer corner of the eye, and translucent face powder, applied gently with a velour puff, set the eye make-up and foundation. Then a clothes colour was added – a small dot of bright green powder eye shadow, to match the green of the sweater,

was blended to the outer edge of the eye. And a yellow powder eye shadow, which complimented the dress, was used to highlight the inner half of the lid and browbone. The eyes were finished with dark brown mascara.

A touch of peach blusher gave the cheeks warmth, and lips were coloured orange.

Make-Up Used:
Ivory foundation
Pale yellow cream shadow on lid
Khaki-green eye pencil in socket
Grey pencil definition to outer corner of eye
Bright green powder shadow to outer edge of eye
Yellow highlighter to inner lid and browbone
Dark brown mascara
Peach blusher
Orange lipstick

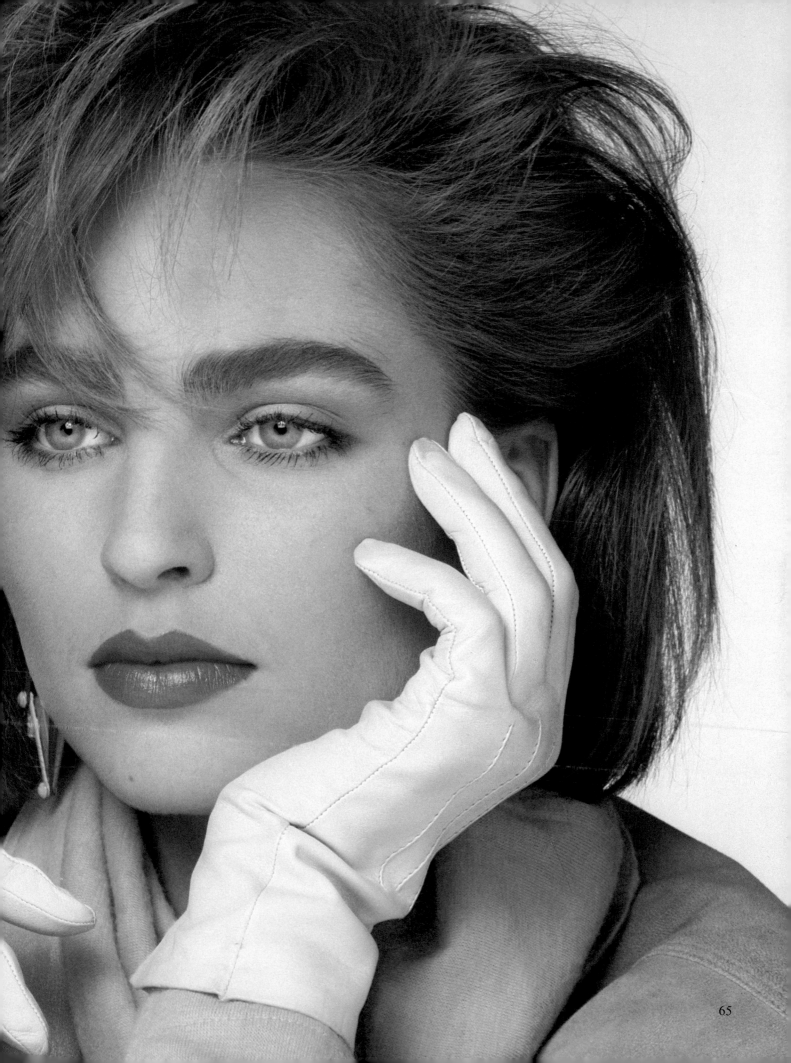

UNDERSTATED MAKE-UP

Bold make-up is fun for younger faces, but if you're over thirty you need subtlety – an understated make-up is softer, and very flattering.

It's more important than ever for *you* to choose a foundation that is a perfect skin match. Skin begins to look paler as you get older, so too dark or heavy a shade is instantly false and ageing. Finish your base at the jawline, not right down your neck, and choose a light texture that blends away to nothing.

For eyes, keep to taupe, brown or soft shades of grey – no hard blues or greens, which can look garish. Go for navy or dark brown mascara rather than black, and comb it out well to make the most of your lashes.

Go easy on the blusher, but wear enough to give 'life' to the skin without looking too 'made-up'. Lips look good either with clear bright colours – well defined, or with soft neutral browny-pinks – for an up-to-date look.

Light beige foundation was applied and blended well into the jawline. Eyes were shaded with silver grey powder shadow over the lid, and taupe powder shadow blended into the socket line for extra depth, and round the outer corner of the eye. All the definition they needed was provided by a fine line of navy eyeliner at the base of the lashes, and by navy blue mascara.

Cheeks were dusted lightly with very soft beige-pink blusher, and lips were filled in softly with browny-pink lipstick.

Make-Up Used:
Light beige foundation
Silver grey powder eye shadow on lid
Taupe powder eye shadow in socket
Navy blue eyeliner
Navy blue mascara
Beige-pink blusher
Browny-pink lipstick

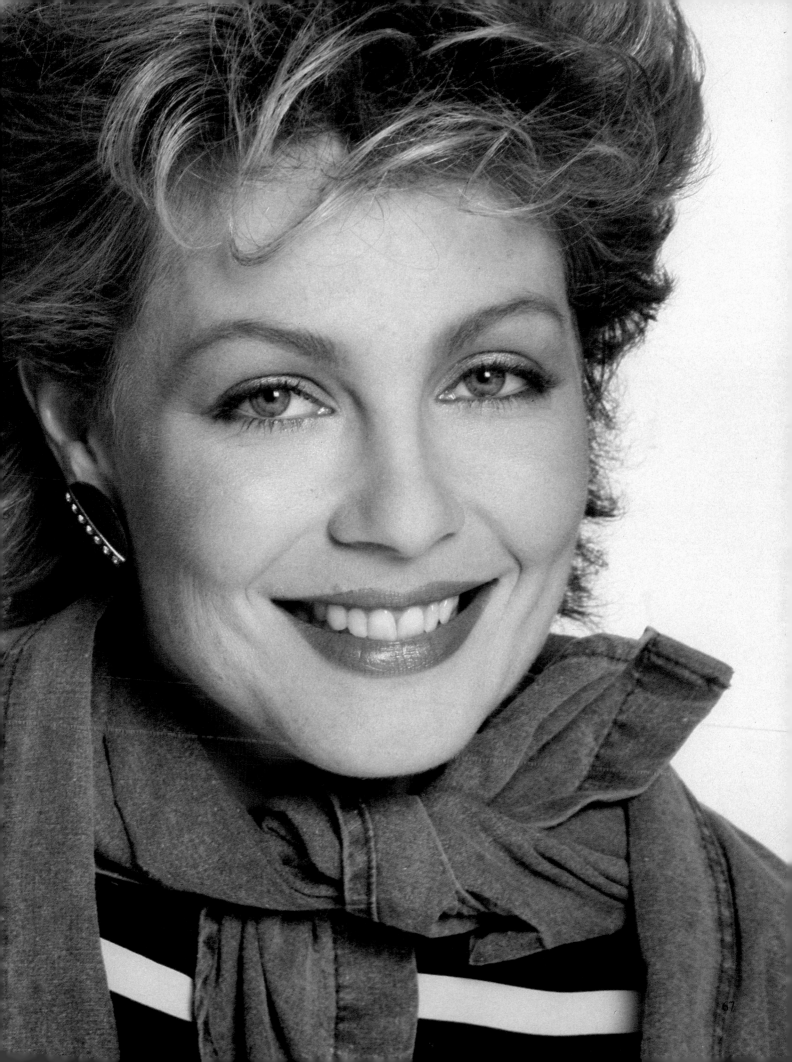

A PARTY PIECE

Party time means make-up can be fun and different – colours can clash; nails go brash; and eyelashes can be unreal!

Now that you've got a special occasion, take time to decorate your nails. Go stripey, with a pattern of red and pink polish together. Or, for a more simple effect, paint your nails with one colour but leave your half-moons unpainted.

Don't feel that lips, nails, and clothes always have to match. It's fine to mix up contrasting shades – as I did here, with bright fuchsia dress, pale pink mouth, and scarlet nails.

False eyelashes are also fun; as long as you stick them on to stay!

The model's party look started with a light ivory liquid base blended away down her neck. Then a series of blacks and greys gave her eyes a smoky evening feel. Black kohl pencil was smudged and blended carefully with a brush all around the eye shape. The whole face was powdered with loose transparent powder, and pale bluey-pink blusher added a glow to the cheeks. Matt grey eye shadow lightened the upper lid, and was blended away towards the brow, then black cake eyeliner was used to re-define the eyes. Long false lashes were the final party touch – with mascara, of course.

The lips were outlined with a pink pencil and filled in with a pale pink lipstick.

Make-Up Used:
Light ivory foundation
Black kohl pencil around the eye
Bluey-pink blusher
Matt grey eye shadow on lid
Black cake eyeliner
False eyelashes
Black mascara
Pink lip pencil
Pale pink lipstick

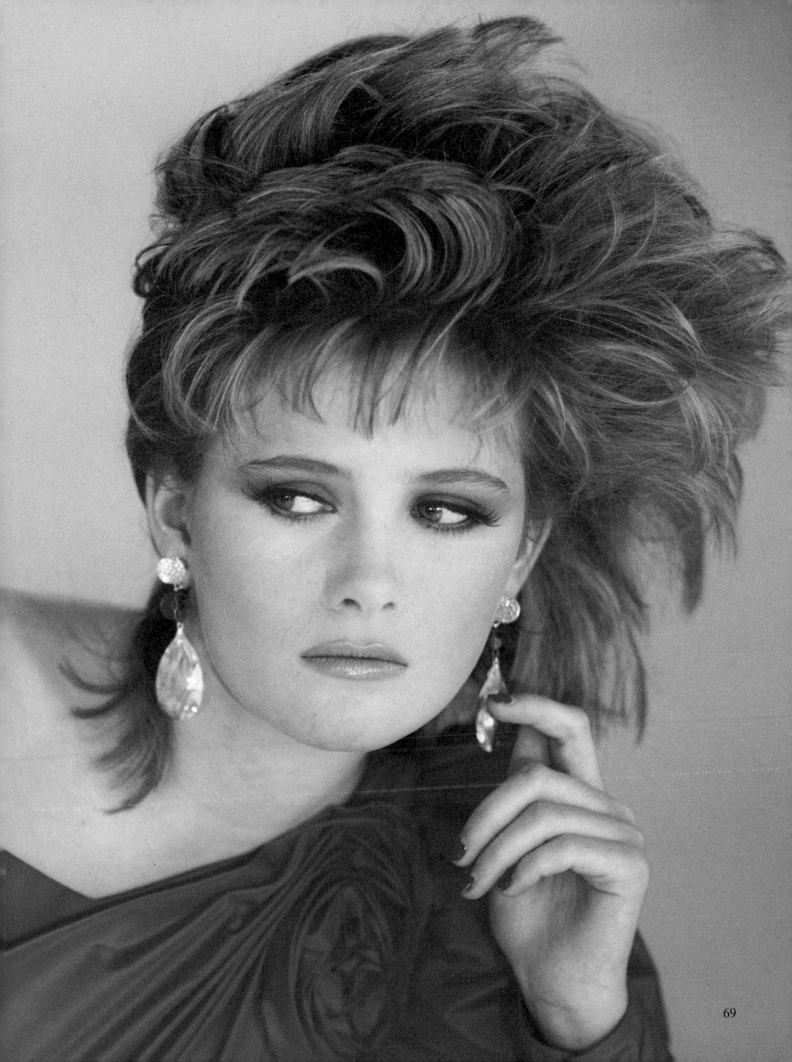

LOOK FOR DAY

Matt and shiny make-ups can be
combined to give light and shade to your
face. But how do you know where
to put what? The clever way to change
a day look to one for night is to turn
on the shine. On this page I'll show you
the day look – then turn over the
page for the night-time version. It has the
same colour tones, but with shaders
and shine added in the right places.

*For a day look you need a matt finish. I started
with a cream-textured, honey-toned foundation,
topped with transparent face powder.*

*A matt-finish peachy-brown powder eye
shadow was brushed all over the upper lid and
blended well to be smooth, with no patches.
Peachy-brown blusher was fluffed over the
cheeks.*

*The eyes were defined beneath the lower lashes
with light brown eye pencil, blended again to
leave no harsh lines. Then reddish-brown
mascara emphasised the eye shape. If you prefer,
you can ring the changes with coloured mascaras
– blue or green, for example, to emphasise your
own eye colour.*

*Finally the lips were outlined and filled in with
a browny-pink lip pencil, smoothed into the lips
with a fingertip to prevent harsh edges.
Alternatively use a lip-coloured lipstick.*

Make-Up Used:
*Honey-toned foundation
Peachy-brown powder eye
shadow on lid
Peachy-brown blusher
Light brown eye pencil beneath
lower lashes
Red-brown mascara
Browny-pink lip pencil*

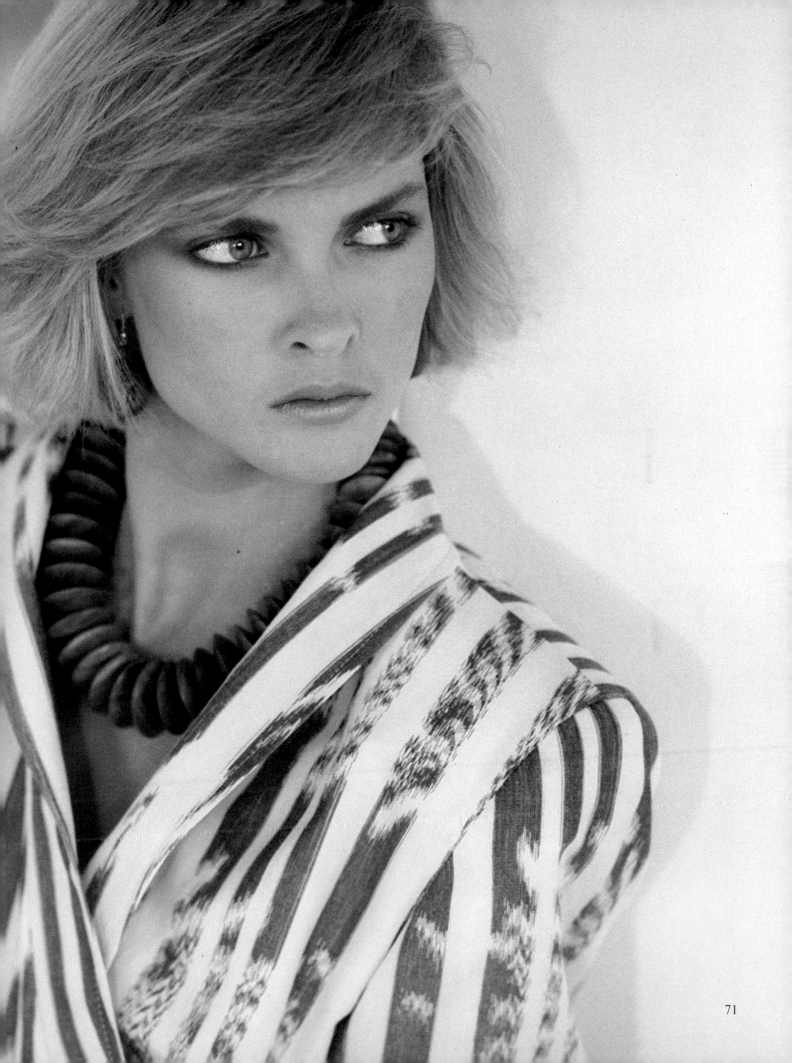

LOOK FOR NIGHT

The basic day make-up was turned into an evening look by emphasising the eyes, lips and cheekbones with shiny cosmetics. Usually any cosmetic with pearl or glitter incorporated in it can be used to add evening sparkle to your regular make-up. Although I have left the previous eye make-up on it is a good idea to cleanse your face thoroughly and re-apply your foundation before going out in the evening.

I used the same honey-toned foundation for the evening look, but instead of powdering the whole face, powder was applied only to the central area – forehead, nose, sides of nose, and chin. The natural gleam was left to shine through on the cheekbones and additional shine was

brushed on in the form of a silver-pink face highlighter. Extra blush was also added to the cheeks for an evening glow.

The eyes were emphasised with a dark grey powder eye shadow brushed into the socket and swept around the outer corners of the eye. A strong silvery highlight was blended over the centre of the lid and a little brushed beneath the browbone. Two coats of navy blue mascara were applied to top and bottom lashes.

A very fine line of face highlighter was used to emphasise the curves of the upper lip, but be careful to blend properly so this doesn't look like a line of perspiration. A clean edge to the lips was achieved by using a lip brush for the deep

pink outline, and the same lip colour was used to fill in. The lipstick was blotted and a shiny gloss was brushed over the top.

Make-Up Used:
Honey-toned foundation
Dark grey powder eye shadow in socket and around outer corner
Silvery highlight on centre lid and browbone
Silver-pink highlight brushed on to cheekbone
Silver-pink highlight on upper lip curves
Pink blusher
Deep pink lipstick and lip gloss

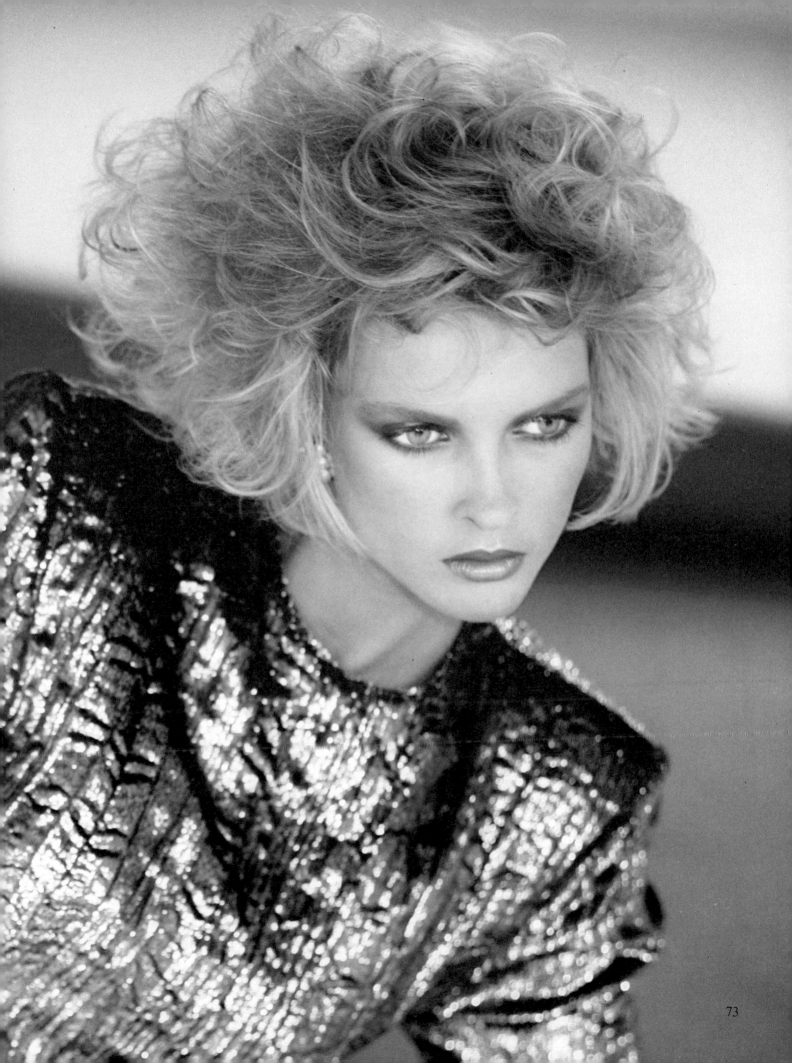

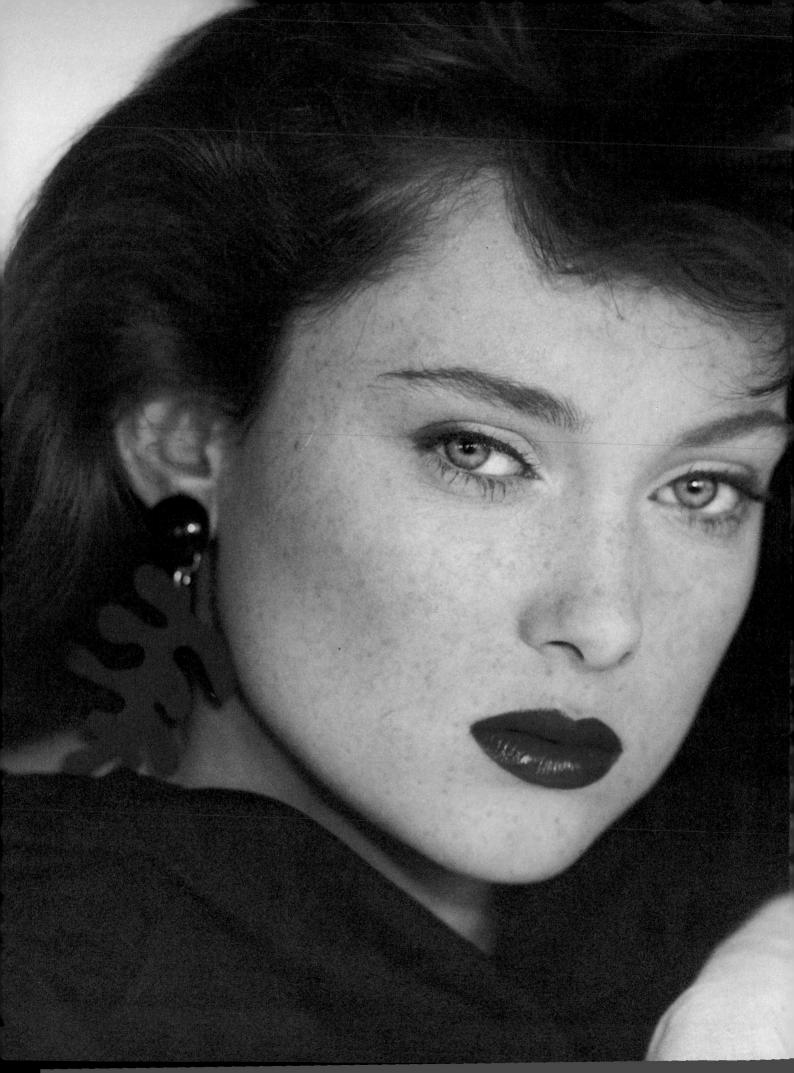

WHAT'S BEST FOR BLACK?

Black clothes make *everyone* look good, whether for simple day wear, sultry evenings, formal affairs or casual get-togethers. But it's a colour that needs careful make-up to show it at its very best.

It's a mistake to try and brighten the look with brash eye colours *and* startling lipstick – the effect is too garish! You need to add just one splash of colour – *either* a bold slick of shadow on eyes, *or* a luscious lipstick on lips. Then add blusher to warm your cheeks. Resist the temptation to put colour into your face with a dark foundation – skin tones should always be skin-coloured!

Here I've chosen to team subtle eyes with bold lips – a look that French and Italian women wear to perfection when making black look so chic!

A pale beige, transparent foundation was used on our model; thin enough to allow her natural freckles to show through, while covering any slight discolouration in the general skin tone. Her eye shape was emphasised with a grey-green pencil line in the socket. This was well blended with a brush, and the face lightly powdered. A creamy-yellow highlighter brushed on to her eyelid gave shape to the eye, together with a very fine brown pencil outline at the outer corners to add length. With the addition of a coat of ginger mascara, the whole effect was one of very understated eyes.

The face was finished with a dusting of pale peach blush, and then a scarlet red lipstick. The lips were outlined with red pencil first, then filled in with a brush.

Make-Up Used:
Pale beige foundation
Grey-green eye pencil in socket
Creamy-yellow highlighter on lid
Brown eye pencil at outer corner
Ginger mascara
Pale peach blusher
Scarlet-red lipstick

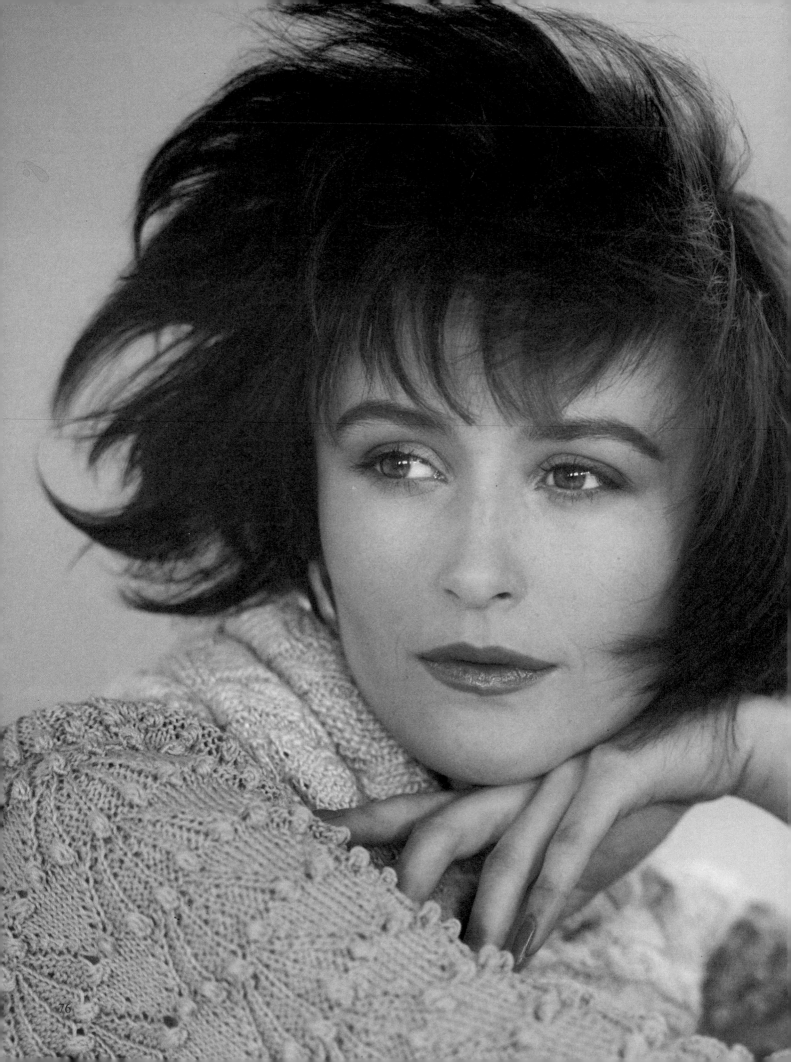

QUICK FACE

In a hurry? Here's a quick, no-fuss, one-colour make-up that will see you through when time is short, but good looks still matter! The right colour, tools and techniques make everything super fast!

Choose a natural skin-tone colour for your eyes – bronzes, pinks and peaches are good, and need less careful blending than brighter colours. Cosmetic pencils are fastest – they can be used on eyes, cheeks *and* lips. You'll also need a darker shade of powder eye shadow, a highlighter, mascara, face powder and lip gloss.

The look will suit almost any age group, and be suitable for day or evening wear – depending on how much make-up you decide to put on your eyes. Here I've used shades of rose and browny pink that match our model's sweaters, but you could just as easily choose peaches and peachy browns for a one-colour make-up.

Liquid foundation glides on quickly – it was applied with a sponge for speedy blending. Dull pink eye pencil emphasised the eyes – drawn close along the lash line and blended away up to the brow. A touch of pink highlight was stroked across the browbone, and on the lid over the top of the eye colour, after it has been powdered. The same dull pink eye pencil was used on the cheeks as blusher. A light dusting of translucent powder set the make-up, and brown mascara finished the eyes. Then the same versatile pink pencil was used to colour the lips – topped with a slightly pearlised rose-pink lip gloss.

Make-Up Used:
Light beige liquid foundation
Dull pink eye pencil on lid
Light pink highlighter on browbone and lid
Brown mascara
Dull pink eye pencil as blusher and lip colour
Rose pink lip gloss

WHAT'S RIGHT FOR WHITE?

When summer's here the whole world wants to wear white – it's a fashion colour that will never die! It can be bright and brash, or coolly sophisticated, but it's always eye-catching! So how do you get your make-up to match? Bright eye colours could overpower the subtlety of white. So avoid blues, greens and bold shadows, go for neutral tones – grey, russet, brown, etc.

White throws the face into contrast and reflects light up on to the face. You may think it is 'draining' you of all your colour, but don't be tempted to try and *add* colour to your face with a dark foundation – this is the most common mistake. Keep your skin make-up skin-toned – then add a little blush for colour, and lipstick. The whole spectrum of lip shades, from bright scarlet, to flesh-coloured pink can look right for white.

The foundation was a pale honey colour which matched our model's skin tone exactly. Her eyes were outlined lightly with dark brown eye pencil, and her whole face powdered with transparent face powder. Coppery-brown powder eye shadow was applied to the eyelid for depth without heaviness. A touch of cream-coloured powder eye shadow highlighted the browbone, and the eyes were finished with brown mascara.

Blusher wasn't necessary here because of the natural warmth of the skin, but if you do feel very pale, a coral, peach or pink blush fluffed on to the cheeks will enliven your face. Finish with pale peach lipstick.

Make-Up Used:
Honey foundation
Dark brown eye pencil around eyes
Coppery-brown powder eye shadow on lid
Cream-coloured powder highlighter on browbone
Brown mascara
Pale peach lipstick

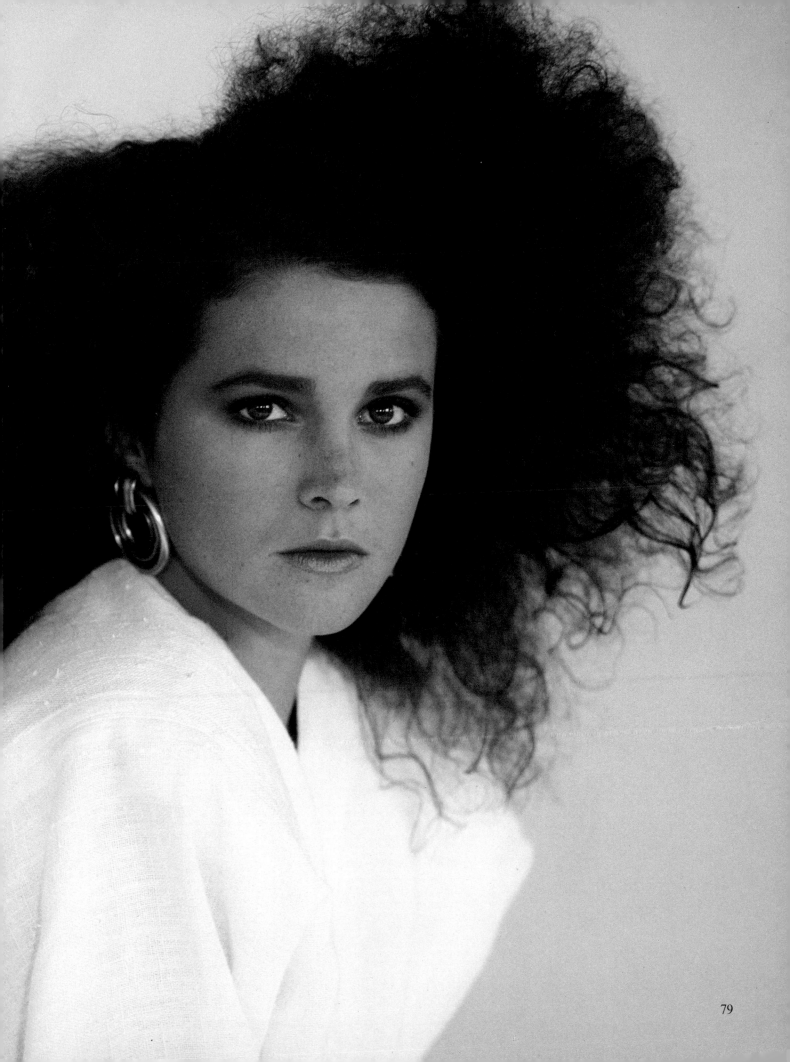

INDEX

A

Acne 11, 13, 18
Air conditioning: skin protection 18
Allergic skin 10–11, 12
Aloe vera 12
Anti-perspirants 21
Astringents 10, 13

B

Bath salts 21
Black clothes, make-up for 75
Blackheads 11, 13, 14
Blushers 33, 37
Body care 21
Body lotion 21
Body massage (in salons) 27
Bubble baths 21
Bunions 25

C

Carbohydrates (in diet) 20
Central heating: skin protection 18
Cheese 20
Clay-based face masks 16
Cleansers, skin 9–10
Cleansing 12–13
Collagen 12
Concealers 33
Corns 25
Cucumber face mask 16
Cuticles, care of 22

D

Daytime, make-up for 29, 70
Deodorants 21
Diet, healthy 20
Dust: effect on skin 18

E

Elastin 12
Electrolysis 27
Evenings, make-up for 29, 37, 72
Eyebrows: darkening 27
    pencils for 27, 38
    plucking 14, 26–7
Eyelashes, dyeing 27
Eyeliners 38
Eyes: care of 57
    make-up 38
    make-up brushes 38
    make-up for blue eyes 40–3
    make-up for brown eyes 44–7
    make-up for green eyes 48–51
    make-up for grey eyes 52–5
    moisturisers 10, 12–13
    removing make-up 10, 57
    shapes 38
Eye shadow 38
Exercise 20–1
Exfoliation 16, 18, 21

F

Faces, make-up for different
        shapes:
    long 36, 37
    round 35, 37
    square 34, 37
Facials, home 14

Fatty foods, cutting down on 20
Feet, care of 25
Fibre (in diet) 20
Fingers, stained 22
Flannels 10
Flower waters 10
Foundations 30–1
Fresheners, skin 10
Fruit (in diet) 20
Fruit face masks 16

G

Gel face masks 16
Gooseflesh, preventing 21

H

Hands: care of 22
    exercises for 22
Herbal face masks 16
Honey (in beauty treatments) 12
Honey and oatmeal face mask 16
Hypo-allergenic ranges 10, 12, 31

J

Jojoba 12

L

Lanolin 11
Lemon (as astringent) 12
Lips: altering shape of 61, 62–3
    making up 61–3
    protecting against the elements 18
Lipsticks, choosing colours 61

M

Making up in a hurry 77
Manicuring nails 22
Margarine 20
Mascara 38
Masks, face 16
Massage, skin 14
Mineral water (as skin toner) 10
Moisturisers 10, 12, 13
    for harsh conditions 18
Moisturising 12–13

N

Nail polish, applying 22
    for a party 68
Nails, manicuring 22
Natural ingredients in products 12
Neck, moisturisers for 12
'Night' cream 12

O

Oil-based face masks 16
Older faces, make-up for 66

P

Parties, make-up for 68
Pedicure 25
Perfume (as irritant) 11, 12
Perspiration problems 21
Pores, open 10, 33
Powder, face 33
Protein (in diet) 20

R

Rain, effect of 18

Roughage (in diet) 20

S

Salons, beauty 27
Sebaceous glands 10
Skin: care routine 12–13 (*see also*
        Body care)
    cleansers 9–10, 12–13
    combination 10–11
    dry 10–11
    fresheners 10
    moisturisers 10, 12
    oily 10–11
    protection for city living 18
    protection against the sun 18
    protection against the weather 18
    sensitive 10–11
    toners and tonics 10
    types 10–11
Soap, use of 9, 10, 13, 21
Spectacles 57
Stress, relieving 21
Sugar, cutting down on 20
Sun, protection against 18
Suntan creams 18
Swimming 21

T

Tiredness, relieving 21
Tissues 10
Toenails, care of 25
Toners, skin 10
Tonics, skin 10
Toning 12–13
T-zone 10, 11

V

Vegetable face masks 16
Vegetables (in diet) 20
Veins, broken 11
Verrucae 25
Vitamins: in creams 12
    in food 20, 22, 57

W

Walking: barefoot 25
    for exercise 21
Water (as skin toner) 10
Wheatgerm (in beauty
        treatments) 12
White clothes, make-up for 78
Wrinkles 12

**PHOTOGRAPHIC
ACKNOWLEDGMENTS
The author and publishers would like to
thank the following for providing
clothes, jewellery and equipment for
photography:**

Marks and Spencer; Browns 40–41, 52–3, 58–9,
70–71, 72–3; Butler and Wilson (jewellery) 4,
28–9, 52–3, 66–7, 72–3, 78–9; Chloe 28–9, 40–41;
Conrans 14–15, 16–17; Descamps 14–15, 16–17;
Detail 64–5; Edena and Lena 76–7; Harvey Nichols
70–71; Maxfield Parrish 64–5; Monty Don
(jewellery) cover, 52–3, 68–9, 74–5; Murray
Arbeid 68–9; Patricia Roberts cover; Pilot 48–9;
Pineapple 64–5; P.X. 58–9; Scotch House 48–9;
Verace 44–5, 74–5, 78–9; Victor Edlstein 4; Wendy
Dagworthy 58–9; Yves Saint Laurent 44–5 (jewel-
lery) 48–9.